BECOMING WELL
Again

by

The Rev. Dr. Robert E. Stover

DEDICATION

This book is dedicated to the physicians, nurses, and staff with whom I have worked over the years. All proceeds will be given to medical research.

TABLE *of* CONTENTS

INTRODUCTION

I am a chaplain in four hospitals and I believe what I have learned in this ministry can help you become well again. God made us to be healthy in body, mind and spirit. In this book I propose that faith in God and in Jesus has a positive effect on the healing processes of our body, mind and spirit which maintains our health.

I will also propose the role of stress in producing illness. Negative feelings like doubt, fear, anxiety, helplessness, and anger hinder healing and sometimes cause illness. On the other hand, positive attitudes such as confidence, hopefulness, and empowerment enable us to approach any illness with a perspective that promotes healing.

Throughout this book there will be references to the role of the medical community and a lifestyle that helps prevent illness. Towering over all is the importance of faith in God in becoming well again. The health of a person depends on the harmonious relations among the parts of a person's personality.

God created us in His image and breathed into us the breath of life. God also formed a doctor within us who provides the necessary chemicals and healing processes that sustain us in health and wholeness. Medical and psychological physicians are God's agents to aid the doctor within us to help our bodies maintain homeostasis.

The mind and the spirit are essentials of the whole person together with the body. The mind and the spirit have a direct influence on the body's capacity to produce or withhold these "natural healing powers." Negative emotions like fear, anxiety, hostility, envy, and worry can produce sickness. Positive emotions like faith, hope, love, courage, joy, and laughter help produce healing and wellness.

When sickness comes, each person has the responsibility for his or her healing by entering into a partnership with God and His servants: doctors, nurses, hospital staff, family, and friends. Our search for wellness encompasses the use of all God's resources: natural, medical and supernatural. One of the hospitals where I serve as chaplain has this mission statement: "We are pioneers in improving the way we care for people's health: encompassing mind, body, and soul."-Tahoe Pacific Hospital.

Throughout this book I affirm and illustrate how faith in God and in medical personnel greatly affects the health and wholeness of the person. All methods of healing, whether ancient or modern, whether labeled religious or psychological or medical have one supreme aim: the restoration of health. What follows in this book is an elaboration and illustration of the assertions made in this introduction.

CHAPTER 1

The Agonizing Question of Illness

Many people ask when they are ill: "Why did this happen to me? What have I done to deserve this?" For one who believes that God is good, sickness appears contrary to a loving God. It is important to understand that God does not will sickness, but rather He can bring some good out of the sickness. John Sanford in his book, Healing and Wholeness, writes: "Greatness seems to be born out of pain, conflict, and struggle and not out of peace, unless it is the 'the peace that passes all understanding,' that ecstatic sense of oneness that comes as a gift of God to the struggling soul."[1]

In the midst of suffering the important question is not "Why am I suffering?" but, "What good can I do with my suffering?" Our faith does not protect or exempt us from the common lot of humanity, i.e. peril, injury, disease, grief, and death. When we link our suffering with God's suffering love revealed on the Cross, the fellowship with a suffering, loving God is possible. Our suffering can serve some great purpose both in blessing others and in glorifying God.

If we recognize that sometimes God heals and that sometimes He doesn't and that the refusal to heal is in the interests of a higher good, then we can accept the refusal as being as much the gift of God as the healing. The refusal may mean a higher compliment than the healing, for in the latter case God refuses us on the basis that the refusal is His faith in our spiritual strength.[1]

---

1   John Sanford, Healing And Wholeness, (John Knox Press/Louisville, Kentucky-1992) page 8

When people ask me to pray that they be healed, I always reply that I will, provided that in case God should not heal, they will not lose faith in Him. For I feel that it is more important that we keep our faith than that we keep our health. With the faith intact even though healing is denied, we are ready for a second alternative, namely, that we can employ the infirmity in the purposes of a higher good.

When a storm strikes an eagle, it sets his wings in such a way that the air currents send him above the storm by their very fury. The set of the wings does it! So God gives us an inner set of the spirit by which one rises above these calamities by the very fury of the calamities themselves. Job is an excellent example. In spite of all the calamities that fell upon him, he kept his faith in God. Job said, "Though He slay me, yet I will trust Him." Job 13:15 His story ends with greater blessings bestowed upon him by God.

St. Gregory of Nyssa once declared, "The soul who is troubled is near to God." It is not peace of mind that brings us wholeness, but struggle and conflict that brings enlightenment to the soul. Deep inside each organism is something that knows what that organism's true nature and life goal are. It is as though there is within each person an Inner Center that knows what constitutes health. When our conscious personality becomes related to this inner Center, the whole person begins to emerge to bring us wholeness. The movement towards health may look more like a crucifixion than adaptation and peace of mind.

To be healthy is to become whole. We can say that the truly healthy person is the one who is involved in the lifelong process of becoming a whole person. Wholeness is harmony among the physical body, the mind, and the spirit. Becoming whole does not mean being perfect but being completed. Wholeness involves growth and often happiness. It is often painful, but it is never boring.

It is not getting out of life what we want, but wholeness is the development and purification of the soul. People often refer to the process as being tested by fire. All of us encounter circumstances where not to be vulnerable to suffering would mean that we did not care about our life and other peoples' lives.

A mother who lost her baby requested to see a chaplain. Her first words to me were: "God gave me a baby girl and then He took her away from me!" She was both angry and crying. I had to fight back my tears in order to minister to her. I replied that the illness took your baby and God received your baby back into His loving arms. She looked surprised and asked me to pray for her baby which I did. She stopped crying and apparently stopped being angry at God but pleased with the idea that her daughter was now in heaven with God her Heavenly Father.

Soren Kierkegaard, the great Danish philosopher, insisted that Christian suffering is to be distinguished from misfortune by the fact that it is voluntary. We willingly take on the pain and suffering of others. As he suggested, we should not confuse losing one's shirt on the stock exchange with giving one's money to feed the poor-though our check book balance may turn out to be the same.

To agree that Christian suffering is voluntary does not mean that the Gospel invites us to run out in search of self-torture. Instead, suffering is met and accepted in connection with faithfulness to aims that we wholeheartedly espouse. We may have additional suffering as the result of our dedication to our purpose in life. To live is not only to live for our own welfare but also for the welfare of others. An example would be those volunteers who responded to the needs of the victims of Hurricane Sandy even at the risk of their own lives.

Dr. Albert Schweitzer, a medical doctor, turned down the opportunity for a prominent career as a physician to offer his life and skills for the suffering people of Africa. Likewise, Dr. Martin Luther King, Jr. saw the sufferings and injustices that the black people were enduring in the United States and so dedicated his life to change the laws that permitted and encouraged such prejudice through loving non-violent resistance to those laws. He was arrested and placed in jail and finally paid the price with his life. Dr. King learned the technique of loving non-violence resistance from Mahatma Ganhdi who won the freedom of the people of India from Great Britain.

We believe that pain is an evil thing, and we seek to reduce it whenever and wherever we can. But no one can live long without confronting the fact that love and suffering go together. Mothers out of love for their baby endure the pain of childbirth and the risk of death. No one can serve in the military without the risk of injury or death out of love for his/her country.

God blesses me as a hospital chaplain where I hear the voices of both love and suffering. Being admitted to the hospital is a pivotal point in one's life. What results from the experience varies: for some it is a time of personal transformation and growth; for others it is a waste of time marked by bitter resentment against the hospital and/or God.

What makes the difference? Where is the sense of the sacred found within the walls of suffering, pain and death? It is extremely helpful to the patient's family and friends to know what happens to the person who enters the hospital. In the attempt to regain one's health through hospitalization one is initiated in a 'rite of passage.' The concept of initiation may be a helpful means of understanding the crises of hospitalization. It may also be a means of bringing suffering and wholeness into creative dialogue and of enabling the patient to assume a more self-conscious, participatory role in the healing process.

The process of initiation takes place in three phases: separation, betwixt and between, and transformation. In the first stage of separation, the patient temporarily relinquishes control over his life. He or she will be placing himself in the hands of others: separating himself from family, community, work, and many other aspects of his life that are familiar and routine.

Upon admission he must answer many questions about his life. Once in his room he exchanges his clothes for a non-descript hospital gown. He is encouraged to send all jewelry and other valuables home with relatives. A name tag with a number to identify the patient and the name of his doctor is secured to his wrist. Hospital schedules and routines are imposed on him, and his freedom is restricted. Roommate selection, room temperature, noise level, fresh air, and visits from nurses and doctors are not within his control.

The second stage consists of lab tests, examinations, diagnostic work-ups, scans, cultures, X-rays, and consultations. With each procedure the patient becomes nervous over the level of intrusiveness which each test may bring. The anxiety of the patient increases with every loss of privacy. The uncertainty of his future, which is hanging in the result of each test, bear upon the ultimate questions that he is raising: concerning the length of his life and possible death.

A patient asked me to anoint him with oil and to bring him Holy Communion. Then he asked, "You're not giving me Last Rites are you?" I replied that I was giving him the sacrament of the sick which provides God's help to make him well. "That's what I want," he remarked.

The patient finds himself reflecting on his life: recalling memories that are warm and reassuring as well as painful and guilt-ridden. What the person has taken for granted, he now craves for and promises himself that once he gets out of the hospital, he will appreciate the simpler experiences of life. Family, friends, flowers, and cards serve as a strong bond with life that exists outside of the hospital. He realizes a clearer awareness of several values: life is precious, and life is finite.

The beginning of a transformation may be brewing within the patient. He came through the wilderness of tests; he felt the unknown in which he questions God's goodness. He has weathered the storm and is wiser and stronger. The doctor informs him that he can go home. The patient removes his hospital gown and puts on his own clothes. The nurse removes his wrist band and returns his valuables. He is no longer a patient.

The third stage of transformation rarely happens in the hospital. However, for those who do undergo a transformation there may come a new purpose for their life and certainly a sense of gratitude for the gift of healing and health. One realizes that he has come through this crisis with a good outcome. The word crisis means danger and opportunity.

I was called by the nurse in charge saying that a patient wanted to see me. She said that she awakened him that morning and told him that the surgeon was going to amputate his right leg in a few hours. Since I had seen him several days before, he requested that I come to see him. When I arrived in his room, he said he was very upset even though he knew that an amputation was possible. I listened to him and then asked if he would like for me to pray for him. He emphatically said yes. After I was finished praying that God would use the skill of the surgeon to bring about a successful surgery and give him peace and healing, I noticed he was much calmer. When I came to see him the next day, he greeted me with a smile. He asked me if I would bring him a Bible which I did. The danger of his surgery was past and the crisis brought a transformation in his spirit. He lost a leg, but he gained a relationship with God.

One of the women in our Cancer Support Group, which I co-lead, told the group that she would rather have cancer and God than not to have cancer without God. She too is going through a transformation because of her illness.

Why do the innocent suffer? There is no adequate answer in this life. We all agree that children do not deserve to be born with deformities and disabilities. One father said to me, "I am angry at God that this disease has come upon my daughter. Let me be the one who is sick. She has done nothing wrong."

Not long ago I was called to the emergency room to meet with the parents of a two-year old who had just died of aspiration from her vomit. The mother told me that they were not church-going people, but she needed the assurance that her child was in heaven. The child's father said he used to go to church and went through Confirmation but had not gone to church for 15 years.

They were grieving deeply and reaching out for God's assurance that their child was with Him in heaven. I shared scriptures that tell of Jesus taking children up into His arms and blessing them. He also told the people that those of childlike faith are in God's Kingdom. In response to the father's request, I baptized the child as an outward sign that she was with the Lord in His Heavenly Kingdom. The words from the scriptures and the baptism help ease their emotional and spiritual pain.

The hospital is a place of life and death. Most people begin their life there. 73% of the persons who die, die in a hospital. As the numbers go, the average time that a patient spends in the hospital is very small. It seems long because of the intensity of the experience often far outweighs the number of days spent there.

For some, hospitalization is a time of celebration. Healthy babies are born; flowers and balloons fill the room with joy. Broken bones are replaced or they mend on their own. Pain is relieved through medication. Hope abounds. God's goodness is praised.

For others, hospitalization is a time of sadness and remorse. Babies are delivered dead or soon die after birth. Feared symptoms are confirmed. Breasts are amputated and arms and legs also. Hope is dashed to pieces. Uncertainty is the outcome for others. Doctors say, "We're going to send you home and carefully monitor those symptoms. Right now we just don't know what to do." Some patients get answers they don't want; some get answers they want, and others get no answers at all.

At a deeper level, sickness often makes strange what had been familiar. Our body doesn't seem the same. What over the years was a trusted, dependable companion is now a stranger. In illness one is not often at home in one's body and one's emotions. The energy demands of illness often make one physically and emotionally drained. Raw feelings of terror, guilt, rage, and confusion surge to the surface in great intensity.

Uncontrollable sobbing and tortuous self-recriminations are common expressions of illness. Such powerful emotions can be unnerving and embarrassing to the patient and to loved ones. Too often nothing seems to be under control–internally and externally–in sickness. At such times the understanding and compassion of the medical team and family can be very re-assuring.

The Reverend Robert Davis, once a pastor of a large Miami church, wrote in his book, <u>My Journey Into Alzheimer's</u>,[2] of the subtle changes within what had been a brilliant mind-bizarre symptoms and behavior patterns. At the age of 53 after months of tests, the doctor finally gave him the results-Alzheimer's, permanent and irreversible. His doctor said to him, "I wish I could tell you that it's cancer."

The book is extremely inspiring and informative, written by a man who helped others to the end of his life–using his last lucid thoughts to share his walk of faith into this dreaded disease. "My spiritual life was most miserable. I could not read the Bible. I could not pray as I wanted because my emotions were dead and cut off. There was no feedback from God. As I tried to sleep, only blackness and misery came, misery so terrible that I could not drop off to sleep. Nighttime was horrible. My mind could not rest and grow calm but instead raced relentlessly, thinking dreadful thoughts of despair. Invariably I lay there terrified by a darkness I could not understand.

My mind also raced about, grasping for the comfort of the Savior whom I knew and loved for emotional peace that He could give me, but finding nothing. If I cannot find fellowship and joy again, what will happen to my professional life? I cannot lead Christ's Church into light and truth when I am full of darkness. Why would God allow this to happen at the height of my effectiveness in the ministry? I groaned out "My God, why?" We are deeply indebted that Reverend Davis shared his journey into mental darkness. For Mr. Davis his disease took away his ability to pray.. What is the role of prayer in the healing process? We will address that question later in the book. We all suffer from a terminal illness called life. Illness is the expression of our physical, emotional, and spiritual limitations. When you accept illness as a fact of life, you are really acknowledging that you are human. As a human being we have limitations, and one of those limitations is that you can become ill at any point in your life.

Disease brings us awareness of our limitations. According to the Bible, the serpent told Adam and Eve: "You will not surely die. God knows that in the day you eat thereof your eyes will be opened, and you

---

2   Robert Davis, <u>My Journey Into Alzheimer's Disease</u>,(Tyndale House Publishers, Inc./ Wheaton, I page 10

will be like God: knowing good and evil." Genesis 3:4-5 The limitations of life close in on us until we reach death.

The hope that wholeness brings comes from faith in a Lord who offers us in this limited life a new life that will not die. Even when disease or death finally takes our biological life, we move on into eternal life. So God enables us to say yes: to childhood, to youth, to young adult life, to middle age, to senior years, to retirement and finally to death.

One day when I was visiting a patient with Alzheimer's disease, I found her tossing her head from side to side, with her husband sitting next to her bed holding her hand. In my clinical training I learned that one of the last functions of the brain to go in this disease is your memory of music. Music is one of the first things we learn as a child. Since she had been a church organist for many years, I asked him what her favorite hymn is. He said, "Amazing Grace". I began singing the hymn. To the astonishment of us both, she stopped moving her head and looked at me singing the hymn with me. After we were done singing, the husband remarked that was the first time she had said anything in months. I urged the husband that when she went home that he or someone else sings hymns with her. I wonder why that hymn was still vibrant in her brain when all the rest was disappearing.

For those who are fortunate to live to old age we come to know that old age foreshadows death. In the last analysis all anxiety is reduced to anxiety about death. Proof of this is the large number of stories in which a man freed from the fear of death is seen to be free of all other fears. He has not fear of anyone or anything; no one can overcome him even by killing him. All people attempt to repress this fear. We are aware that someday we will die. We can postpone the day by maintaining our health, but eventually we die.

Who can deny that the end of life is death? Now the meaning of death is the religious question par excellence. Does there exist something other than the visible world in which we are enclosed from birth to death? My old age has meaning. I can live through it with my gaze still fixed before me and not behind me trying to live in the past, because I am on my way to a destination beyond death.

Whatever project we may be working on in old age, our eyes also need to be fixed beyond death. We may not be able to complete our present project for whatever reason, but one thing is sure: we will die. Death is the moment of truth which upsets all our vain categories. There is a physical factor in our anxiety over death which reminds us that we are not pure spirits despite all our high soaring doctrines of eternal life. It is this animal weakness, and not our spiritual side, which is the root of the question that challenges the goodness of God.

Pain and suffering can be educational for us. They may serve as a warning that keeps us from ways of living that produce pain and suffering. In our cancer support group, nearly everyone had smoked in his or her lifetime. Now that they have cancer, they have stopped smoking. Pain and suffering can also bring new meaning to our life. Several members of the cancer group volunteer in our hospital helping other cancer patients through their difficult times. People who have lost loved ones are comforted by family members and friends who come to see them, telephone them, and send cards and flowers. "Blessed are those who mourn for they shall be comforted." Matthew 5:4.

"We may learn and grow from suffering. Life is not so much what happens to us as what happens in us."[3] We can look for the creative and redemptive note in suffering. It is possible through the grace of God that suffering can be transformed into creative, redemptive power. Isaiah the prophet, in his description of the suffering servant, has presented in poetic form the figure of one who took upon himself the suffering of others and was able to transform it into power that helps others. The perfect example is Christ upon the cross.

Others have been able by the grace of God to use their own suffering and new insight gained from their experiences to help others. Several years ago, I met a thirty-one year old patient who was paralyzed from his neck to the bottom of his feet. He was in a car accident in which he hit a pole that left him paralyzed. When I walked into his room, he gave me a cheerful hello. He was in the hospital because of a bed sore. I remarked about his cheerful spirit. He told me he was drunk when the accident occurred. "God has blessed me by showing me His love in Christ, and I am so glad that I was found by Him." He also told me that God is using him to reach high school students by speaking at assemblies when he shows them what can happen when you mix alcohol and driving. God has given him a radiant personality to serve as a testimony to God's love.

The typical New Testament attitude towards suffering is: "How can this be used to further God's purpose in the world?" For the Christian then the question of suffering comes to this: "How can I use my suffering to advance the Kingdom of God?" In the midst of suffering

---

3   Wallace Viets-My God Why? (Abingdon Press/Nashville-1966) page 7

one can complain and give up, or one can accept the suffering in the confidence that God will sustain you using the suffering to help others.

Some people believe that their suffering is a punishment from God. That attitude adds spiritual suffering to their plight. Job's neighbors and even children treated him with scorn unthinkable. Job is overwhelmed by his suffering and privation. He ends up on the village dump throwing ashes over his boils and scratching his sores, weighed down with their judgment. They accuse him of hiding his sins. His wife leaves him and recommends that he curse God and die. Unquestionably the reaction of Job's neighbors, children, and wife represents the attitude of people in those days towards anyone struck down by adversity and serious illness. These were signs that a person had lost favor with God through his wickedness. But Job maintains his innocence and in the end was justified by God.

The relationship between a faith in a loving God and the healing of the body, mind, and soul is a direct one. Love is the answer to suffering as revealed in the life of Christ and in His followers. Love is also the basis for modern medicine. The medical community treats all sufferers equally. It is non-judgmental.

Although some illnesses are caused by one's neglect of a healthy style of living, not all of them can be blamed on the actions of the sick person. There are diseases caused by genetic heredity. Medical research is discovering some of the answers to genetic causes. There is a lady in our cancer support group that received a stem cell transplant from a young military man. The result was that she was healed of her cancer. The transplant took place six years ago.

So the healing may be of the body in this life or healing through death when we are clothed with a spiritual body free of illness. In either case, God removes the disease or removes us from the disease. Jesus did not fall into the error of believing that all diseases are caused by sin. In Luke 13:2-5 people came to Jesus to tell Him about the Galileans whose blood the Roman governor, Pilate, had mingled with their sacrifices. Jesus responded: "Do you think these Galileans were greater sinners than any other Galilean? They were not greater sinners." Jesus clearly stated that those who suffer tragedy are no more sinful than other people.

In another instance the disciples questioned Jesus about the man born blind. Jesus tells them that neither this man nor his parents sinned…he was born blind so that the works of God might be displayed in him. Jesus then healed him of his blindness. Modern medicine looks to genetics and chemical imbalance as the source of much illness. In addition to these causes, I believe that faith in God strengthens our body, mind, and spirit.

Many people today assume that illness borne properly makes for a better and stronger person in all areas of their life. This is uncomfortably close to the idea that sickness endured will bring cleansing to the ill person. One must be stoic in the face of sickness. Holding to that belief, then it is wrong to relieve the pain and to strive for health. In that view, one perceives God as enjoying a very human anger against people and will love them only when they are morally good. Sickness then becomes a weapon by which God reaches out in anger at humans, because they have overstepped the bounds he has set for them. Jesus completely rejects this view of illness.

The coming of Jesus denies the view that sickness is caused by sin, and because of that sin, God in His anger sends sickness to the sinner. Jesus' healing ministry embodies the exact antithesis of this idea. He did not inquire whether the person was good or bad before He healed him. He loved people just as they were and wanted to help them out of their misery whatever the cause. If sin had caused the misery, Jesus' attitude was that once this person is healed he will have a greater opportunity to come to his senses. As long as he is sick, it is difficult for the person to come into a loving relationship with God.

Jesus gave no hint of sitting back to wait for suffering to teach a person a lesson and thus bring him back into faith in God. Jesus knew that healing and love could accomplish God's will in humans far better than punishment. God is more interested in creating wholeness in people rather than using them to satisfy His divine anger.

Nuclear energy can be used for saving lives or destroying life in war. I was a naval officer in World War II. Our ship was anchored near the island on which the city of Hiroshima stands. It was just two months after the city was devastated. I took a motor launch over to the island and stood in the midst of the rubble and disintegrated ashes of human beings. It is estimated that somewhere between 70,000 and 80,000 persons were killed either immediately or afterwards from the radiation.

When I was doing my graduate work at Princeton Theological Seminary, I walked by Dr. Albert Einstein twice but never spoke to him because he always had his head bowed, and I figured he was in deep thought. I heard him speak once. Here was the man who discovered $E=mc^2$. The formula was always there, but it took Dr. Einstein's research to discover it. Since Hiroshima, nuclear energy is used to save lives through medical tests that diagnose diseases. Likewise, we have the freedom of choice of how we will live a healthy life or disregard the laws of health.

An important lesson I have learned about health is that one may be cured of an illness but not necessarily healed. The opposite is also true. One may not be cured of a disease but is healed in his mind and soul. Or a person can be both cured and healed from an illness and thus reach a higher state of health and wholeness.

Don Murdock of Laity Lodge in Texas tells of a person who was cured of cancer after a five-year intense treatment. For the next ten years the patient continued to grow bitter in his mind and spirit because he had lost a very promising business during the years of treatment. His rancor alienated his children and his wife. His marriage ended in a divorce.

A mental patient who was suffering from a heart disease and a sexually transmitted disease came to know the Lord's love and forgiveness. The last years of her life were a journey toward wholeness. Her faith in God enabled her to re-create the brokenness of her life into a mosaic of courage, trust, hope, faith, love, and beauty. She had come to realize that she was a child of God of infinite value. A priest who had reviewed the healings of Lourdes said that people are mistaken if they think that "miracles produce faith." Quite the opposite is true: "Faith produces miracles."

Disease reminds us of our limitations which we often unsuccessfully try to deny. Recently a twenty year old male patient who was now a quadriplegic told me that he jumped out of a four story window thinking he was to have a soft landing in the tree. He missed the tree and landed on the ground beneath him. He shared that he had done a very foolish thing. He was holding on to the hope that the surgeon remarked that he had a slim chance of regaining the use of his limbs. As a cardiologist once told me, the thinking part of our brain doesn't reach its full development until the age of twenty two. The patient realized too late to acknowledge his limitations. It takes a lot of living to realize our limitations. Those limitations close in on us when we finally reach death.

In an unfinished world, faith in God enables science to discover curative methods of medicine, surgery, and self-care such as: exercise, diet, and meditation. Our culture focuses on the symptoms of illness, whereas Jesus put the major emphasis on the attitude taken toward the illness. The essence of health, as Jesus saw it, had less to do with the absence of symptoms than with an inner state of wholeness out of which physical health emerges. "This inner state of mind is independent of organic conditions and is not dependent on an absence of suffering. Indeed, suffering itself may contribute to an inner sense of wholeness and peace. Whereas our culture tends to avoid suffering at almost any cost, the New Testament faith, developing as it did out of the crucifixion followed by the resurrection, insists that something very redemptive can emerge out of suffering."4 There is a sense in which suffering is just as much a part of life as is pleasure. Rightly [4]understood, suffering contributes far more to life than pleasure. Ralph Waldo Emerson wrote, "We acquire strength by the obstacles we have overcome." Those who are fortunate to live to old age eventually come to know that old age means that death is near.

I was called to the bedside of a patient who was dying, and I asked him what he would like me to do for him. He replied: "I would like peace before I die." So I repeated the promise of the Lord: "My Peace I give to you, not as the world gives, give I unto you. Let not your heart be troubled neither let it be afraid." John 14:27

Robert Browning penned these words:

> "Then, welcome each rebuff
>
> That turns earth's smoothness rough,
>
> Each sting that bids nor sit nor stand but go!"
>
> (From "Rabbi Ben Ezra")

God has work to do to finish His creation of man and suffering plays a major role. Victor Frankl gives a large place to suffering in his work. Like Carl Jung, he sees the attempt at avoiding suffering as being a sort of neurotic pattern. Frankl writes that suffering and trouble belong to life as much as fate and death. None of these can be subtracted from life without destroying life's meaning. To subtract trouble, death, fate, and suffering from life would mean stripping life of its form and shape. Only under the hammer blows of fate, in the white heat of suffering, does life gain shape and form."

Because Victor Frankl was a Jew, he was interred in a Nazi concentration camp. He noticed that the prisoners who survived were

---

4   E. Stanley Jones- The Word Became Flesh, (Abingdon/Nashville-1963) page 3

those who shared their meager rations with other prisoners. Frankl explained the reason for their survival was that they had found a higher meaning to their life, i.e. giving food to those who did not have enough. There is always something we can give to others from our life.

In the conviction that suffering belongs to life and can be used creatively to complete and to discover the meaning of life, Frankl underscores the conviction of Jesus. The Christian faith has always been concerned with the elimination of human suffering, as innumerable hospitals erected under Christian auspices all over the world indicate, but the condition of physical health is only part of the concern. The larger concern centers on one's response to sickness. In a similar way Frankl's approach is one that looks more at the attitude of the sufferer than at the conditions of suffering.

Since the tendency in medical circles is to focus attention on the symptoms, the underlying attitude of the patient is lost sight of. Frankl asserts that many symptoms are the direct results of unhealthy attitudes, and that often relief can be accomplished by changing the attitude of patient rather than the symptoms.

In this understanding the question asked by Jesus of the Bethesda cripple is valid: "Do you want to be healed?" The implied question is: "How do you look on your illness? Is it a means of getting lots of attention? How does your illness affect your attitude toward life?" The question of Jesus, "Do you want to be well?" directed attention not to the man's illness but rather to his outlook on life. Whereas the invalid talked in terms of the help that others never gave him, the result was that he lost hope. Jesus put the emphasis on his attitude about himself. Concerned for so long with how others could help him, the invalid had overlooked how he might help himself.

Jesus directs the man's attention to the future rather than to the past. What is important is the adoption of a new attitude which gives the person the power to handle the symptoms. It is important to take note that when attention is focused on attitudes, then there is never a situation which cannot be helped. I like Goethe's saying, "There is no predicament that we cannot ennoble either by doing or by enduring."

Health for the crippled man meant only recovery from the symptoms. But Jesus opened up the whole subject of the meaning of his illness. Meaning can be found in the very attitude that is taken toward suffering. The very way in which a man faces his destiny creates, for him, the opportunity of realizing values and hence of finding a meaning in life. Jesus knew that there was unfinished work to be accomplished in this man's life for a complete healing.

Martin Gray, another survivor of the Holocaust, writes of his life in his book, For Those I Loved. He relates how, after the Holocaust, he rebuilt his life, became successful, married and raised a family. Life seemed good after the horrors of the concentration camp. Then one day his wife and children were killed when a forest fire ravaged their home in the south of France. People urged him to demand an inquiry into what caused the fire, but instead, he chose to put his resources into a movement to protect nature from future fires. He said that an investigation would focus only on the past, on issues of pain and sorrow and blame. He wanted to focus on the future. An inquiry would set him against other people: "Was someone negligent?" "Whose fault was it?" Life, he concluded, has to be lived for something, not just against something.

The German theologian, Dorothy Soelle, asks whose side we thought God was on in the concentration camps: the murderers' side or the victims' side? In her book, Suffering, she suggests that the most important questions we can ask about suffering is whom does it serve? Does our suffering serve God or the devil; the cause of becoming alive and more complete in an unfinished world; or being morally paralyzed? Not where does the tragedy come from but where does it lead is the real issue.

"The Word became flesh." John 1:14. This is the great divide of all other religions in which the Word became a word, a philosophy, a list of morals, a system, a technique; but for all time and for all men everywhere, "the Word became flesh".[5] The idea became a fact and a reality. The logical consequence of God becoming a human being is that God suffers and knows pain and death in the life of Jesus Christ."[5] God knows what it is to suffer at the hands of evil people.

The Christian faith is God taking His own medicine. He deliberately took our weaknesses and sorrows at a deep cost to Himself. It is the supreme example of love to be found in the universe. God finished the work of His Kingdom in His Son Jesus Christ, and now He invites us to discover that finished work of healing.

---

5   E. Stanley Jones-The Word Became Flesh, (Abingdon/Nashville-1963) page 3

A poet wrote:

> He who formed our frame
>
> Has made man a whole;
>
> And how the health of the body
>
> Depends upon the soul.

What is the Christian view of health? It includes good health when possible; spiritual healing always; prevention of illness and personal responsibility for maintaining whatever health is possible for self; and conscious acceptance of aging and dying. It is a vision that includes the body as the temple of the Lord.[6]

"I sometimes feel that I just want to give up -that fighting to recover is too hard and is taking too long."[6] Each time a new diagnosed cancer patient comes to our support group, he or she expresses amazement that he must now think about the possibility of dying. Our culture has an obsession with issues of health and youthful beauty. Over 10% of our nation's gross national product relates to maintaining a youthful appearance.

The cost of disappointing the gods of health is a sickly life: loss of self-esteem and premature death as people find themselves vacillating between feelings of omnipotence and impotence. Wholeness is ultimately a matter of spiritual connection with God whether our body is healthy or sick.

I was called to the bedside of a young man who requested to see a chaplain. In a very depressed tone of voice he said, "I've lost my connection to God." I prayed for the renewal of his connection with God and for his physical health. In a more relaxed voice he thanked me for coming and for praying for him.

---

6   Herbert Benson-<u>Timeless Healing</u>, (Scribner/New York-1996) page 12

CHAPTER 2

How Does God Heal?

One way God heals is through the knowledge and skill of the doctor. He is God's agent of healing. The doctor treats the patient, but it is God who heals. The doctor clears away the obstructions to allow our body's natural healing powers to function properly. All the healing forces reside in our body, ready and waiting to restore our body's balance.

Dr. William Osler, considered one of the greatest physicians and surgeons who ever lived, believed that his success as a healer was due to aspects of personality and behavior that brought forth the patient's faith in the effectiveness of the treatment and to the care and comfort provided by good nursing care. When Dr. Osler used the expression "faith healing", he referred to the psychological influences that set in motion the restorative mechanisms of self–healing. The instant he entered the sick room the patient felt better.

The art of healing seemed to surround his physical body like an aura. It was not often the treatment but his presence that cured. Francis Peabody's famous remark, "The secret of the care of the patient is in caring for the patient." This is another way of saying that there is a miraculous moment when the very presence of the doctor is the most effective part of the treatment.

The physician is more than a prescriber of medications but the symbol of all that is transferable from one human being to another. We will not live forever in this life, but we persist in the notion that the physician possesses the science and artistry that will provide us with endless deferrals of our death. He seems to be in command of those sources where the secrets of life are stored. To be able to listen to the beat and rhythm of the heart and draw meaning from its slightest variations; to be able to take a tiny droplet of blood and perceive its vital balances and to convert electrical markings into precise knowledge of the body's complexities–all these represent science to the doctor, but to the patient they are powers that come from Gods.

Two personal examples: A number of years ago I went to see my doctor about a sore throat. He patted me on my leg and said, "Chaplain Stover, we're going to get you well." His confidence aroused my faith in him and in his words. I distinctly remember I began feeling better at that moment.

Recently I went for my annual check-up with my family doctor. He had a medical student with him that day and asked her to listen to my heart. After she had listened, she said that she heard a heart murmur. The doctor confirmed her finding and then asked her what kind of a murmur is it. She mimicked the sound and the doctor said that it was not that kind. Then he imitated the sound and told her to listen to my heart again. She did and said she could hear the murmur just the way the doctor described it. I was amazed at the teaching which took place in my presence and with my body. It increased my confidence in my doctor.

In their preparation to become a physician, students study long hours learning about the human body and how the parts of it work together to maintain health. Students also study and observe the effects of various drugs that promote healing and the negative side effects of those same drugs. Then there is the skillful art and knowledge of the surgeon to correct broken bones and organs of the human body. In the hospital where I serve as chaplain, I see many students in the various stages of their training, and how hard they work to acquire their credentials as a doctor.

God heals through psychology. You can create a climate of disease or health by your negative or positive attitudes. Dr. Thomas Hora, a psychiatrist, wrote that malicious thoughts about others are probably the psychological basis of malignant diseases. Malicious thoughts are thoughts that enjoy the misfortune of others. "How does an individual become malicious-by practicing unloving thoughts about others; finding fault with others and blaming them? Pretty soon one begins to enjoy other people's misfortune. This way one gets caught up in a quagmire of malice…It is, therefore, to cleanse ourselves of all malicious thoughts under any circumstances, no matter what the provocation."[7]

---

7   Thomas Hora-Dialogues In Meta-psychiatry, (The Seabury Press/New York – 1977) page 25

Jesus said, "Love your enemies." Some think this is foolishness, but I believe it is profound wisdom. Nobody can hurt us as much as we ourselves with our own thoughts. We can be our greatest enemy. The best way to be blessed whether sick or healthy is to be a blessing to the others. Also when we say to others: "God bless you!" we receive a blessing in return whether the other person returns the blessing or not. In my hospital work I always bless the person when I leave his room.

One day I walked into a patient's room and introduced myself to a male patient. He said, "Chaplain, I don't believe in God." I said to myself: "Well, I'm not going to talk about God with this man." I noticed on my patient sheet that he was the age of World War II period. I asked him if he had served in the war. He told me that he had been in the Navy. I said that I too was in the Navy during World War II. We had an enjoyable time sharing some of our experiences from the war. When I left the room I said: "God bless you." He replied to my surprise: "God bless you, too." We made a connection!

Our attitudes in life affect our behaviors and our vulnerability to illness or they contribute to our health. We have a choice. It's as though there are two attorneys in our mind: one gathering evidence for the view-"life is awful" and the other gathering evidence for the view-"life is awfully nice!" You're the judge who can rule out any evidence you want. Your decision is final. One ruling leads to frustration, fear, worry and sickness. The other leads to more joy, happiness, peace, and health. Your decision often is final. However, you have the freedom to choose the view that promotes health.

The Christian faith and its healing powers have much to do with human behavior. One's behavior can make a great difference as to whether one is sick or well. Another member of our cancer support group died from lung cancer. She had smoked for forty-five years and stopped when she was diagnosed with cancer. She did not blame God for her cancer but rather sought the help and support of a loving God through her faith and her church.

Dr. Herbert Benson, professor of Medicine at Harvard Medical School, wrote in the foreword of his book, Timeless Healing: "My hope is that this book will help you appreciate the power of your beliefs so that you can embrace life and the meaning of your life for the fullest measure of health."[8] Dr. Benson noticed that his patients' progress and recoveries often seemed to hinge upon their spirit and their will to

---

8   Herbert Benson-Timeless Healing, (Scribner/New York-1996 page-12

live. He believes that the human mind and one's spiritual beliefs have physical manifestations.

After his junior year in college, Dr. Benson served as a merchant marine seaman. He informed his shipmates that he was planning to become a doctor, and some of them came to him when they felt sick. He gave them vitamin pills and they improved rapidly after taking the pills and seeing him. When the doctor tells you that you are sick, then that label has a negative effect on one's psyche and physical health. All of us project our intense desire for wellness onto the doctor and the medicine we take. It is known in the medical community as the "placebo effect."

Dr. Benson calls the placebo effect "remembered wellness." It is human nature to color our reality with hopes, emotions, philosophies, and convictions. Because beliefs and emotions are ephemeral and imperceptible, western medicine has largely assumed that their effects are not physical or measurable. Western medicine is more interested in the mechanical operations of the body than the effects of the mind and the spirit upon the body. However, today Western medicine is taking a new look of effects of the mind and spirit upon the body.

He believes that beliefs do matter and that they have physical repercussions. He also believes that the human spirit is relevant and influential in the treatment and prevention of illness. He has found that there is no greater healing force than the power of the individual to care for and cure himself. Jesus said, "You shall love the Lord your God with all heart and mind… and your neighbor as you love yourself." Matthew 19:37-38 Notice that Jesus includes loving and caring for yourself as you are called to love your neighbor.

For Dr. Benson the ideal model for medicine is a three-legged stool. One leg is surgery and procedures; the second is drugs and the third is self-care. The most neglected part of healing is self-care. Our source of healing that is timeless is our physical endowment from the day we are born. The three components of "remembered wellness" are:

1. Belief and expectancy on the part of the patient.

2. Belief and expectancy on the part of the caregiver.

3. Belief and expectancies generated by a relationship between the patient and the caregiver.

We learn in childhood how to please others in order to gain a reward. In medicine this pleasing is called the placebo effect, from a Latin root meaning: "I shall be pleasing or acceptable." Most health professionals and patients are eager to please one another: the former by being friendly, hopeful, and confident in the therapies being recommended and the latter by getting better; by complying with instructions; by getting and by reporting improvements in health.

One study concerning the effect of the doctor's words upon the health of the patient revealed that 64% of the patients who heard good news from the doctor got better within two weeks. Only 39% of the patients who did not hear good news from the doctor got better within two weeks. The weight of the doctor's words was proven all the more powerful, because statistically there was little or no difference between those who received prescriptions and those who didn't.

I saw this in the remarks of a member of our cancer support group. He shared with the group that he decided to go to the top physician who specialized in treating the kind of disease he had. He was so pleased with his doctor that he told the group: "He spent an hour with me on the phone. It felt good to get that kind of attention from and access to such a doctor.

It is evident that a positive, supportive approach is an essential part of the healer's personality. No matter how precise the surgery, studies show that you will recover your health if your surgeon is upbeat, confident, and kind. In every incident of remembered wellness, the catalyst is belief in your doctor. The belief may be your own or a composite of your life's experiences. Belief can be instilled in you by your caregiver. A prominent physician concluded that it isn't the circumstances of your life that are critical but your attitude toward these circumstances that seals your fate. The faith or faithlessness that governs our life affects our health.

Studies have also shown that patients who consistently follow their doctor's orders, believing that doing so would make them well, were twice as likely to recover from a serious illness. Much of the success that the medical profession achieves is not due to anything doctors do or dispense that is inherently healing. We can really attribute the healing to the "doctor within" or our immune system. Our beliefs make a powerful difference in our physical health.

Our soul also plays a significant part in our getting well. Many who are sick have their sickness rooted in a mal-adjustment of their soul to

God. It is not so much a mal-adjustment of the body to the physical environment or the mind to true thoughts. Rather it is the longing for renewed health and vigor that causes the body to respond to the cravings of the soul, sometimes in dramatic ways and at other times subtly.

A patient who came through her surgery with flying colors told me that as she was being taken to surgery, she kept saying to herself: "Be still my soul. God is with you." It is the physician's responsibility to encourage patients to observe good nutrition, to engage in regular exercise, and to maintain hope that the medicine or surgery will result in good health.

"Another important component in our understanding of 'remembered wellness' is the brain's priority established in us even before we are born. This priority is to survive, the propensity which we call 'the will-to-live.' We come into the world with some factory-installed elements called neurosignatures already instilled in our brains. The inborn wiring is determined by our genes and by the contributions of the egg and sperm at the moment of our conception."[9]

Here is a remarkable truth: the brain is malleable and changes constantly, millisecond after millisecond, according to our life's experiences. Our brain constantly recruits new nerve cells and activation patterns to handle its daily inputs: the cereal you eat at breakfast, a smile from a newborn, your rainy commute and the deadlines and quotas expected of you at work. The minutiae of our lives are always absorbed and evaluated with our brain modifying itself to handle whatever threats our lifestyle entails.

So not only is the brain the world's most efficient repository, the efficiency and speed of which has yet to be mimicked completely by any computer. The brain is the trampoline from which springs all action and thought. We are also endowed with survival instincts. The brain is its own artist, chemist and engineer. It is constantly remaking and reconstituting itself. Isn't that amazing? We are at this very moment a very different organism from the one we were a few seconds ago and the one that will be seconds from now. The decision-making structures of our brain direct all this traffic, not only relying on tried and true routes of nerve cell activation but designing new combinations of nerve cells and neurotransmitters to aid our survival and to help us learn new things. What a wonderful thing our brain is!

9　Herbert Benson-Timeless Healing,(Scribner/New York-1996) page 88

But you may be asking: "Where does faith in God fit into this marvelous body and brain of ours? Faith is a positive emotion. Faith in the Ultimate Being of the universe is the highest form of trust. Faith in Jesus Christ who went about performing good deeds and healing the sick is the ultimate placebo! Faith in the Good Shepherd when we are going through the valley of the shadow of death affects our brain and our heart. When I am called to minister to a dying patient, I always recite the 23rd Psalm. Not only do we remember wellness, but we remember our Creator who knitted this wonderful body in our mother's womb. As we were received into the loving arms of our mother at our birth, so are we received into the loving arms of God at the time of our death. There is no more positive thought than that the Power behind the universe is the One that Jesus revealed in His life, death, and resurrection. We call Him our Great Physician.

All of us have distinct neurosignatures for wellness, for illness, for strength and endurance, and the specifics we associate with all the other activities and situations we have faced in life. Both bad habits and good habits follow previous patterns in the brain to become self-fulfilling prophecies. This is how remembered wellness occurs. When we change our minds or outlook on life, we can do a great deal to improve our health. Nature and nurture are inseparable and interdependent. "O Lord, you have made us for yourself and our hearts are restless until they find their rest in Thee." St. Augustine.

There are times of illness when no remembered wellness or faith in God revive the function of our lungs or keep our heart beating. At such times we need the tools of modern medicine to keep us alive. Too often we take for granted that trauma centers and emergency rooms routinely snatch patients from the clutches of death. Diagnostic tests give us months and even years of prior notice to halt an encroaching disease. Antibiotics and vaccines save us from scourges that imperiled our ancestors and that still continue to imperil much of the world today. We are grateful to modern medicine for extending our life span. However, not all diseases have been eradicated. The multiplicity of different colored wrist bands reminds us that there are many diseases to be conquered.

Medicine has confined its definition of "what we are made of" to cells and bones and not always taking into account the rich gamut of moods and ideas that also affect our health. The Psalmist said, "What is man that You, O Lord, are mindful of him? For you have made him a little lower than the angels, and You have crowned him with glory and honor." Psalm 8:4-5

Throughout human history medicine had to rely on the human spirit and other seemingly mysterious sources of healing. For primitive medicine, the placebo was all there was. Early medicine had many practitioners: priests, healers, sorcerers, medicine men, witch doctors, witches, shamans, midwives, herbalists, physicians, and surgeons who relied exclusively on unproven potions and procedures. The fact that some patients got well had much more to do with the natural course of their disease and with the belief that they were going get well than with the inherent value of the medicine or procedure. Much of the history of medicine is the history of the placebo effect.

God heals through the surrendering of fears, resentments, self-centeredness, guilt, and negative feelings. These emotional feelings and destructive thoughts help produce illness. Galen, Greek physician, born around A. D. 130 said, "He cures most who most are confident." In early medicine the relationship between healer and patient was sacred and mystical in quality. Jesus recognized the importance of this relationship when He said to the woman who reached out to touch his garment, "Your faith has made you well." Mark 5:34

Seneca, the Latin philosopher who lived from about 4 B.C. to 65 A.D., appreciated the role of hope in healing and wrote: "It is part of the cure to wish to be cured." So much of the input to the brain is pessimistic, violent, and anxious. As a result, our body suffers the nasty side effects. It is so important to take a positive outlook on the events of our life that influence our health.

When illness does come, "many people have discovered a way to tap the emotional strengths and spiritual powers available to those who are children of God."[10] Our personal value is at stake when we are unable to work because of sickness. Society measures us by our ability to produce. In our cancer group two middle-age men have retired because they are no longer able to keep up with the demands of their work. In addition to the challenges of their illness, they had to face the loss of their value to their company. Figuratively, they had to retire early at a monetary loss. Now these men place a higher value on "living each day to the fullest" and doing those things they want to do: travel, fish, hunt, etc. while they are still able to do so.

---

10   Vernon J. Bittner-Make Your Illness Count, (Augsburg Publishing House/ Minneapolis 125) page 10

Through surrendering the negatives of life we can be free to establish new relationships. Psychiatry emphasizes that in order to find wholeness we need to experience a new relationship. This is the central theme of the Bible. Because of sin our relationship with God has been broken, and what was whole is now in pieces. Christ offers a new relationship through faith in His healing work. He brings peace to those whose life is in pieces. He makes whole those who are broken.

New life comes from the "experience of acceptance that we have from God and from one another." We call this acceptance, love. It is a new kind of love: agape. It is love for the unacceptable one even with all his faults. "We love Him because He first loved us." 1 John 1:14 A member of our RV camping group was diagnosed with stage four lung cancer. His doctor told him he had about three months to live and to get his affairs in order. He was very depressed about the diagnosis. I called him on the phone and shared the fact that a number in our cancer group were told that they had six or less months to live, but they were still alive two or more years later. I then asked him if he knew God's peace. He said he would like to know that. So I prayed for him that he would accept the gift of peace and wholeness that God was offering him. After the prayer he thanked me and said he felt much better. Several weeks later he was baptized and made whole in his faith in the Lord.

Not long ago a Vietnam War veteran requested to have a chaplain visit him. After I entered his room and introduced myself, he said that he doesn't think God could ever forgive him for the innocent people he killed even though he was ordered to do so. He said that it didn't bother him until about two years ago. Since then, he could not forget it or believe that God could forgive him. I told him that all of us are sinners. I was in World War II and a part of the military forces who had to do what you were commanded to do. That statement created a bond between us. There is no sin that God would not forgive when confessed. I asked him if he would like for me to join him in prayer for God's forgiveness. He said, "Yes, I need it." After the prayer he said he felt much relieved. The next day when I went to visit him, he smiled while thanking me again. His mood of depression had lifted.

Complete retirement from an active life does not seem to be a good way to reach a very old age. Rather it is the act of surrendering those attitudes and habits that destroy life. It is taking on new attitudes that are positive and new habits that enrich life and tend to extend our life. "Dr. Alexander Leaf of Harvard Medical School has made extensive clinical and social observations of very old people in several parts of the world. His studies have led him to suggest that longevity is correlated with a rather frugal diet but of well-balanced composition, vigorous and continued physical activity, and involvement in community affairs to the end of one's life."[11]

Death is not the ultimate tragedy in life. The ultimate tragedy of dying is in an alien and sterile area, separated from the spiritual nourishment that comes from being able to reach out to a loving hand, separated from a desire to experience the things that make life worth living, separated from hope.

A patient in an intensive care unit is provided with everything diagnostically necessary in an emergency--everything except the sense of security and ease that the body needs even more than the clicking surveillance of technology. Such surveillance tends to create a sense of panic, itself one of the multiplier of dis-ease. Many doctors are increasingly aware of the circular paradox of the intensive care unit.

One day the husband of a patient in the intensive care unit was advised that he should approve the removal of his wife's life support. He told the doctor that he would not approve of it until he talked to a chaplain. When the husband and I had privacy to speak, he told me of the situation and would I pray for his wife. I went with him to his wife's bedside and prayed. When I finished, she opened her eyes to his and my amazement! The next day they removed her to a regular unit. That's when the husband called for me again and told me that both he and his wife wanted to be baptized. He knelt by her bed, and I baptized them both. In a few days she was discharged home. God did a wonderful healing there. I believe the husband's faith was stronger than mine that day, and God honored his faith.

Dr. Jerome D. Frank told graduating medical students that any treatment of an illness that does not also minister to the human spirit is grossly deficient. Norman Cousins reported that a British study showing the survival rate of patients with heart disease being treated in an intensive care unit was no higher than the survival of similar patients being treated at home. His interpretation was that the emotional strain of being surrounded by emergency electronic gadgets in an atmosphere of crisis offsets any theoretical technological gain.

---

11   Norman Cousins-Anatomy of an Illness, (Bantam Books/NY-1979) page14

In that same commencement address, Dr. Frank referred to a study of 176 cases of cancer that went into remission without surgery, radiation, and chemotherapy. The question raised by these episodes was whether a powerful factor in those remissions may have been the deep belief by the patients that they were going to recover and their equally deep conviction that their doctors also believe they were going to recover.

Illness may force the sufferer into a dependent relationship with the person who offers to heal him. If trust does not become an important part of this relationship, it is unlikely that healing will occur. Physicians who ignore the importance of the relationship with the sufferer are often those who possess a simplified philosophy about illness-that is, that illness is the enemy which he assaults with all the skill and technology at his command. But the patient may succumb to the treatment, destruction of the immune system, hospital-borne infections, and surgical mistakes.

When I was a student in clinical training at the mental hospital, St. Elizabeths in Washington, DC, the director of the Chaplains' program taught us that psychiatry made the following contributions to getting well again:

1. Concern for the individual and for his unique integrity. With the mass production, extensive activity, and pre-occupation with groups have made it most difficult for us to see people as individuals. The person is lost in the group classification--the heart patient, the cancer patient or the diabetes patient. Jesus started with a person as he was. He would inquire what was troubling him. The difference is that in psychiatry, the patient is not told what to do whereas Jesus said: "Go and wash; take up your bed and walk; go and sin no more." Jesus addressed the negative aspects of the patient's life. Both the psychiatrist and Jesus listened to the sick person and established a new relationship in which the patient is able to confront his past failures in living, deal with his present inadequacies, and plan realistically for the future.

2. The basic drive of the personality is towards health. God has endowed each person with tremendous life-giving resources that inevitably move him in the direction of health. No doctor gives himself the credit for having cured

the patient, for the doctor is well aware of these inner resources and his own limitations. One is aware that God is really the healer. It could be that our own failures in living have tended to dim our faith in God, in the doctor and in others, so that we no longer dare trust the infinite potentialities with which God has endowed us.

The recovered mental patient is "weller than well" according to the late Karl Menninger. By that he means that the state of emotional health to which the patient has been restored is in fact "superior" to what he had considered well before his illness. This also applies to cancer patients who have actively participated in their recovery from cancer. They have a psychological strength, a positive self-concept and a sense of control over their lives that is better than before. They expect things to go well, and they are no longer "victims of life".

Some healthy and vigorous people die almost immediately after being diagnosed as having cancer. Almost all cancer patients think they have been given a death sentence when the doctor first tells them they have cancer. Such patients are often intimidated by the diagnosis and develop a negative expectancy of their ability to survive that they in a short time die. Doctors will say that the patient has given up or has lost the will to live.

On the other hand, other patients keep a positive outlook and have a good recovery. In these cases the medical treatment was very effective being aided by the patient's positive outlook. They equated treatment with regaining health. One patient told me three times: "I'm going to lick this!" The patient's beliefs are powerful determinants in the outcome of their illness.

A positive response toward treatment is a better predictor of the outcome of the disease rather than the severity of the disease. When I was a chaplain at Hollywood Presbyterian Medical Center in Hollywood, California, I met a Japanese patient who was being treated for cancer through radiation. He began failing in health rapidly. He revealed that he associated radiation with the death and destruction of Hiroshima. Even though his doctors explained to him the difference between the irradiation of the atomic bomb and radiation for medical purposes, they were unable to change his unconscious belief, and he died shortly after beginning treatment. It was a self-fulfilling prophecy.

Wally Mozdzierz is blind. Yet he skies the toughest slopes. In an interview he said that he began with the smaller slopes and liked the challenge of the steeper slopes. Gradually he overcame any fear even though he fell at times. His victory over fear and his willingness to learn how to ski enables him to enjoy the health promoting exercise of skiing.

Greg Anderson in his book, The Cancer Conqueror, describes his incredible journey to wellness. He relates how his cancer was the worst negative he had ever had to deal with. Society conditions us to think negatively about cancer. He writes that "the three major untruths we are conditioned to believe about cancer are:

1. Cancer means death.

2. Treatment is ineffective and has bad side effects.

3. Once you contract cancer there is nothing you can do to help yourself.

The truths about these statements are:

1. Cancer may or may not mean death.

2. Treatment is getting more effective and side effects less severe continuously.

3. Once you're diagnosed with cancer there are many things you can do-especially spiritually, physically, psychologically and emotionally to help yourself.

The untruths lead to beliefs that result in despair. There is no power in despair. Truths on the other hand lead to hope. With hope there is significant power."[12]

Even though one may have cancer that person is not cancer! Right in our own bodies is the mortal enemy of cancer cells-our own immune system. It is not that the surgeons, the radiation, the chemotherapy, or other treatments are all-powerful. They themselves can't cure the cancer. No! The truth is that those treatments help the body's immune system heal itself-from within! The medical team is in a support role to the body's own healing power! Remember the doctor within?

Another fear we need to surrender is that we can catch cancer from a cancer patient. I had two types of skin cancers that came from

---

12   Greg Anderson-The Cancer Conqueror, (Word Publishing, Dallas London Sydney Singapore) page-30

spending too much time in the sun when I was young and serving in the Navy in the hot Pacific Islands. A cancer patient shared with me that his daughter-in-law told him she would not be bringing his grandchild to see him, because she didn't want to expose her child to cancer. Her remarks upset him terribly. Many people avoid cancer patients because they think they can "catch" the cancer. Sometimes the doctor conveys to the family that the patient is going to die. They then gather around the patient as though they were attending a funeral. I have seen and felt this response from the patient while visiting the patient.

Other patients associate the chaplain with impending death. They will say to me, "Chaplain, am I that sick?" I reassure them that my visit is to help them get well. They give a sigh of relief. A patient stands a better chance of getting well when the negatives are surrendered to God.

God also heals through the direct intervention of the Holy Spirit. The Word of God has the power to heal through the inspiration of the Holy Spirit upon the spirit of the person who is ill. The very essence of religion is to adjust the mind and the soul to the love of God. God has made us to find our wholeness and health in a vital relationship with Him. The Word is out in the medical profession that religious practice is correlated with health and longevity. I believe healing is bringing the person into a right relationship with the physical, mental, and spiritual laws of God.

Many people experience the power of God's Spirit in Psalm 23. Its power is not chiefly in memorizing the words but rather in thinking the thoughts expressed in the Psalm. Its power lies in the fact that it presents a positive and a hopeful faith approach to life. Psalm 23 gives one a new perspective on life.

Another powerful effect of the Holy Spirit on the body is found in the miraculous work of our immune system. Spontaneous remission of cancer-an all too rare effect-appears to result from sudden immune activation, which demonstrates the potential of the immune system to react against malignant growth, sometimes with such vigor that large masses of tumor tissue dissolve in a matter of hours or days. When this happens, the patient often exclaims that it is a miracle from God.

It is important to know that cells turn malignant constantly and normally the immune system destroys them-our fighter cells. Given the increasing environmental pressures toward malignant transformation, it is important to keep our healing systems in good working order and to know how to reduce cancer risks. A cancer patient must exercise great care in deciding whether or not to use cytotoxic treatment (radiation and chemotherapy) because damage to the immune system may reduce long-term possibility of a curative response. In this world cancer will always be with us until cures are found.

The most important steps we can take to be receptive to prolonging our life are to stop smoking, to reduce our intake of saturated fat in our diet, and to exercise. "People who exercise regularly report that they are generally happier and in a more upbeat mood when they have had a workout. Exercise releases endorphins in the brain which improves our mood and makes us more optimistic."

A healthy body is necessary to living a full life. Since the body is the temple of the Lord, it is critical to care for God's temple. "Faith without works is dead." James 2:20. One could put these words in a new light: faith without work does not produce a healthy body. Exercise is the key to a healthy body at any age and is also one of the leading factors in living to a healthy old age.

"The prescription for a healthy body is exercise, but exercise of a special kind. It needs to be exercise that comprehends the unique requirements of the aging body and that employs strategies to protect and strengthen the body's traditional weak spots. Most exercise programs emphasize the development of muscles: this one –which gets to the muscles eventually- begins with the body's basic building block, connective tissue. The key to aging is what happens to tissue."[13]

Life is limited, and old age is a vivid reminder of that truth. Job also reminds us of this truth: "Man's days are determined; you have decreed the number of his months and have set limits he cannot exceed." Job 14:5 While we are here on earth, God wills for us to live out those days in wholeness of body and spirit.

Joni Eareckson was a victim of a diving accident that left her totally paralyzed from the neck down. Her entire life was changed from a state of vigorous activity and independence to an existence of total helplessness and dependence on others. She has recovered from her depression and is now able to paint with a brush held between her teeth. "I recall so clearly the details of what happened to me on July 30, 1967. It was the beginning of an incredible journey. Oscar Wilde wrote: 'In this world there are only two tragedies. One is not getting what one wants and the other is getting it. To rephrase his thought, I suggest there are likewise only two joys: one is having God answering all your

---

13   Norman Cousins-<u>Anatomy Of An Illness</u>, (Bantam Books/NY-1979) page 14

prayers; the other is not receiving the answer to all your prayers. I believe this because I have found that God knows my needs infinitely better than I know them. He is utterly dependable, no matter which direction our circumstances take us."

Joni said that losing my anger at God made the difference between suicide at seventeen and a life of strong purpose. The very irony of my story suggests the existence of someone designing destinies. God healed her spirit, and she was able to move on with her life as a strong witness to God's love in the midst of tragedy.

Joni found that God never places any real emphasis on the present-except as a preparation for the future. She continues: we know only a limited sense of reality. This doesn't mean that I'm preoccupied with heaven and the hereafter. It just helps me put things into perspective... the only things we can take to heaven with us is our character. Our character is all we have to determine what kind of a being we will be for all eternity. It's what we are that will be tested by fire. Only the qualities of Christ in our character will remain. Joni's physical limitations led to greater health of her spirit. God's Spirit brought His wholeness to her through faith in Jesus Christ, the Divine Physician.

Music is also an agent of God to bring healing as I previously related the story of the woman patient suffering from Alzheimer's and was yet able to respond to music by singing Amazing Grace. In the Bible young David played the harp to soothe the troubled mind of King Saul. The first scientific study of music as a tool of medicine was published in the Medical Record of 1899. It was demonstrated that music could relax a person and help him to fall asleep, but as medicine grew more scientific, many doctors lost interest in music's benefits for health. Many dentists will give the patient a headphone and the opportunity to listen to the style of music the patient likes. The music enables the patient to take his or her mind off the pain of the drilling.

In 1929, as radio became popular, Duke University Hospital made headphones available to all patients. During and shortly after World War 2, veterans' hospitals used music to improve morale among the injured, depressed, and shell-shocked servicemen.

Of course, music is no cure-all, but it can do some very remarkable things for the body and the mind. In a study eighty people who had suffered a heart attack were divided into three groups. One group listened to a 20 minute audiotape of calming music; another practiced breathing and meditation to evoke a sense of calm; and the third group received standard care. The patients in the music and relaxation group showed significant reductions in heart rate and in the level of stress hormones. The patients who listened to music were the least stressed of the three groups.

A member of my church told me that her brother-in-law had Alzheimer's disease and did not speak to anyone for two years. Then one day he attended worship services in the nursing home and sang, to the amazement of the staff, the old gospel hymns. Music affects the brain in its deepest part, especially the music we learned early in life.

Charles Wesley, the great hymn writer, said: "Jesus! The name…Tis life and health and peace." Jesus and health are synonymous. "Jesus sat wearied by the well." John 4:6 It was a healthy weariness from a long morning's walk. He had no mental or emotional or spiritual conflicts within to cause him to be weary. He had health within Himself and He bestowed health to others.

All our diseases cannot be cured in this life, because death is always a part of this life. However, God enables us to use our sicknesses for greater benefits for others and for ourselves. The Apostle Paul prayed three times that his "thorn in the flesh" be taken away. His answer came: "My grace is sufficient for you; my strength is made perfect in weakness." Paul then responds: "I will glory in my infirmities that the power of Christ may rest upon me. Therefore, I take pleasure in infirmities, in reproaches, in needs, in persecution, and in distresses for Christ's sake. For when I am weak, then I am strong." 2 Corinthians 12:9-10 The truth of this passage is that sickness may bring us closer to God who makes us stronger spiritually and sometimes physically than we were ever before.

Physical healing is not the central emphasis in the Christian faith. God is not here to serve us, but we are to serve God whatever degree of health we can have. God gave Paul the promise of His gift not to bear the infirmity but to make something of value from it. Our final cure is our resurrected body. "The God who raised Jesus from the dead will also give new life to your mortal bodies through His indwelling Spirit." Romans 8:11 In other words, the indwelling Spirit of God gives new life to our mortal bodies.

Studies show that humor is an asset to health. In the Old Testament we read: "…God had made me to laugh, so that those who hear will laugh with me…" Genesis 21:6 God has made us so that we are able to laugh and to enjoy good humor which is a very healthy thing to do.

Laughter tones up the whole body along with the fruits of the Spirit: love, joy, peace, kindness, and goodness." Galatians 5:22 Every emotion has some effect on the body, either for good or bad. Laughing is truly good for our health.

When we pray, we sometimes pray for the intervention of God. By all medical standards Andy Delbridge should be dead. He was diagnosed with the most aggressive and dangerous type of brain tumor. His chances of surviving were no more than a few months. Mr. Delbridge put his trust in his doctors and in God. Members of his church prayed for him daily. He and his family asked for divine intervention and prayed for a miracle. "The minute you think that you have no hope you are down for the count. So you've got to think always that there's hope," said Andy. Today Andy is cancer free. The brain tumor is gone along with the growths that appeared near his heart. They simply disappeared without surgery or any other cancer treatment.

Dr. Harold Koenig of the Duke University's Center for Spirituality, Theology and Health says, "There are hundreds and hundreds of scientific studies that show religious people are healthier than those who have no religious faith." Dr. Friedman who treated Delbridge says that faith cannot be ignored. People of faith generally are more optimistic and as a rule lead healthier lives. How do prayer and other spiritual practices influence physical health? Many spiritual paths or belief systems require certain austerities of the devout which are healthful. Mormons, Seventh Day Adventists and Orthodox Jews are commanded to follow specifics rules regarding diet, alcohol, hygiene and other health-related behaviors that are known to favorably impact morbidity and mortality.

The collective aspect of spiritual practices provides social support which has been documented as a potent protective factor against illness. The psychodynamics of religious beliefs can also promote health. For example, rituals such as prayer may trigger a myriad of emotions which in turn may lead to changes in health by positively impacting the immune and cardiovascular systems.

At times the psychodynamics of faith can be indistinguishable from the placebo effect. If one expects God's blessing, it is more likely to occur. It is the hope a believer has that God wants him to be well and that he will get well. Even on the human level, when we know that others want us to get well, we will be more apt to get well. When you are ill and know that others are praying for you or they come to lay hands on you, then your immune system responds to facilitate healing.

It is sometimes forgotten that medicine owes its greatest debt, not to Hippocrates, but to Jesus. Jesus brought to methods and codes the corrective of love without which true healing is rarely possible. In the opening chapters of the Gospel according to Mark, the ministry of Jesus is characterized as threefold: a ministry of preaching, teaching, and healing, and the discussions occasioned by it. Everywhere Jesus went, he functioned as a religious healer. Forty-one personal instances of physical and mental healing are recorded in the four Gospels. In addition, other healings were recorded as "large numbers of people."

It is clear that Jesus sent His disciples out to continue this ministry of healing. It was the direct action of the Holy Spirit working through Jesus' healings. Even Jesus' opponents did not try to contest the fact that Jesus healed but only to cast doubt upon the agency through which He did it. They claimed that He cast out demons by the power of the prince of demons-the devil. Jesus healed because the Spirit of God was working in him. Luke 11:20 When the disciples of John the Baptist came to inquire if Jesus were the Messiah or should they look for another, Jesus replied, "Go back and tell John what you have heard and seen, the blind see again and the lame walk; lepers are cleansed and the deaf hear; the dead are raised to life, and Good News is proclaimed to the poor." Matthew 11:4-5

This affirmation was evidence that Jesus saw Himself as the Messiah. His healings were the sign needed by John to assure him that he had not preached and baptized in vain. The Gospel writers recorded the healings of Jesus to illustrate that through these healing events, the power of God had broken through into our world and that sicknesses were being put to flight.

This attitude of Jesus marks one of the basic differences between Jesus and other healers in ancient cultures. The Greek healing god, Aesculapis, was simply one god among many. Since Jesus saw Himself as the Messiah who represented the essential nature of God, His healings therefore sprang from the nature of God. Sickness was considered the prime evidence of evil in the world.

The word, psychosomatic, is composed of two Greek words: psyche which means soul and soma which refers to the body. Psychosomatic describes an illness that affects both the body and the soul. Thus the whole person is ill. The body and the soul are so intertwined and connected that whatever happens to one affects the other also. A famous doctor said that If you want to avoid a thrombosis, never forget to say your prayers.

A patient who had previously been diagnosed as being anemic had a blood test which proved to be normal. Her doctor asked her if anything out of the ordinary happened in your life since your last visit. The patient said that she had been able to forgive someone against whom I bore a nasty grudge. All at once I felt as if I could at last say yes to life. The end of the bitterness in her heart was the beginning of healing of her illness. An unforgiving person is necessarily an unhealthy person. A discontented person is on the way to becoming a sick person. An embittered person is already ill in mind and will soon be ill in the body.

An ailing and inefficient body can do much to produce a depressed mind and spirit. The great masters of the spiritual life have seen that the best way to injure the spiritual life is to neglect the body. The Christian view of the body is that our body is something that can be offered to God as a living sacrifice. We need to hold on to the truth that no pain, no illness and no suffering are the will of God. The time will come when suffering will no longer be, and God's will be perfectly realized.

The evidence in Scripture for this is overwhelming. It is the dream of the prophets in the Old Testament that there will come a time when no one will say, "I am sick." From the beginning to the end of Jesus' ministry healing is an integral part of His work. Mark 1:39 The way of Jesus was to bring people into a faith relationship with God by the various methods of touching, speaking commands, compassion, and forgiveness in order that the power of God might break through to restore them to wholeness. Jesus' healing ministry is the logical expression of the incarnation: "God so loved the world that He gave His only begotten Son." John 3:16a Jesus loved people, and that's why He healed them.

Faith in Jesus' love for you stimulates the healing forces within you. But what happens to the body when we die? The health of the body is for this life only. Faith in God enhances one's physical health and is limited to this world. Faith in Jesus Christ as God's only begotten Son brings spiritual health forever. Christ's victory over bodily death through His resurrection is the last healing. "For this perishable must put on the imperishable." 1Corinthians 15:53 The ultimate certainty of this earthy life is death. No matter what your diet; no matter how much you exercise; no matter how many vitamins you take or health foods you eat; and no matter how low your cholesterol, death will conqueror you some day in some way.

The most democratic of all experiences in life is that everyone is appointed by God to die. Hebrews 9:2 Death, like an unfinished symphony, leaves fragments of many promising careers and lives. Why is death the enemy of God since it destroys life that God created in our mother's womb? The Bible tells us that neither sin nor pain and neither disease nor death was part of God's original plan for human beings. A Gallup poll showed that the more education and money people had, the less likely they were to believe in hell. Another Gallup poll showed that 66 percent of the general population said they believe in "a heaven where people who have led good lives are eternally rewarded." More people are confident that there is a heaven than those who are concerned about hell. Knowing that Christ overcame death and promises that those who have faith in Him will have eternal life gives one a profound sense of victory over death. In regards to death and life we have a choice. Socrates said to his disciples when he was sentenced to die on the charge that he was corrupting the youth of Athens with his teaching, "I go to die; you remain to live. God alone knows which of us goes the better way." The death of Socrates saved no one, not even himself. Jesus died to save everyone.

Psychologist Hans Selye points out that it is not the crises of life themselves as it is how we cope with them that counts. Our spiritual forces come to our aid when we reach the end of our other resources. A religious faith inspires a way of coping with life that withstands adversity and even the threat of death. The quality of your faith will create the way you meet threatening events of life: hurricanes, tornadoes, war, sickness, and death.

It is in illness that the quality of your trust in God that reveals its influence on all avenues of your life. A small idea of God lends itself to small purposes. It is not God who is inadequate in times of crises, but rather our idea and faith in God is inadequate. J. B. Phillips points out in his book, <u>Your</u> <u>God</u> <u>Is</u> <u>Too</u> <u>Small</u>, that through faith in Christ we are able to cope with whatever life brings. Alcohol Anonymous' first step is to acknowledge one's need for a higher power to overcome addiction to alcohol. For the Christian that higher power is the God and Father of our Lord Jesus Christ.

If we are sure in our own heart and minds that God presides in a universe of law and order, then we will be freed from the idea that we live in a precarious universe where whim operates and where a capricious deity acts against his own loving nature. Faith makes the difference. There is nothing like a serious illness to compel a person to examine life and to discover what shapes his or her values. One can seek to escape the trials of life or seek to develop the skills to face them.

The body can heal itself. Spontaneous healing is not a miracle but a fact of biology. Each day in which we enjoy relatively normal health testifies to the activity of the healing process. Its inestimable value lies not in its ability to produce remissions of disease, but rather in the maintenance of our health through the vicissitudes of daily life. Here is the real opportunity to appreciate the extraordinariness of the ordinary.

Cancer has always been with us. All living organisms are susceptible to it and the more complex the organism, the higher the risk. Our cancer group therapy dog, Lillie, a beautiful white standard poodle, died from brain cancer. All of us loved her, and it was a great loss for everyone. "A great many pressures on the cells push some of them toward malignant transformation. Malignant cells are dangerous, because they do not die when they are supposed to; do not remain in place but metastasize; and do not limit their growth to conform to the general laws that regulate the economies of whole organism."[14]

Science offers three treatments for cancer: surgery, radiation, and chemotherapy. Given the limitations of these treatments, prevention is all important. Even in its earliest stages the presence of cancer represents significant failure of the immune system. When faced with cancer, the question one tries to answer is: Will the damage done to the cancer justify the damage done to the immune system? At the present time there is no absolute and satisfying answer.

Tennyson said it clearly: Old men must die, or the world would grow moldy and would only breed the past again. It is through the eyes of youth that everything is constantly being seen anew and rediscovered with the advantage of knowing what has gone before: it is youth that is not mired in the old ways of approaching the challenges of this imperfect world. Among living creatures, to die and leave the stage is the way of nature--old age is the preparation for departure, the gradual easing out of life that makes its ending more palatable not only for the elderly but for those also to whom they leave the world in trust. If God were good, He would wish to make his creatures perfectly happy, and if God were almighty, He would be able to do what He wished. But the creatures are not happy. Therefore God lacks either goodness or power or both. This is the problem of pain in its simplest form.

---

14   Andrew Weil-Spontaneous Healing, (Ballantine Books/New York- 1995) page-329

In the Bible we are told that all things are possible with God. God has limited Himself in a world of natural order in which there are fixed laws that unfold with casual necessities together with free will, and thus suffering becomes inevitable. As to God's goodness, there is no lack of goodness in God. We are the ones who are evil through the misuse of our free will. The whole point of the Gospel is that Jesus Christ took the pain of our wrong doing both in His spirit and in His body in order that we would be pleasing in God's sight. That is the Good News! It is often through the pain of suffering and illness that we come to see that we need to be made over into a more lovable person.

Nothing unfavorable can ever happen to us but that, in co-operation with God, we can turn it into a spiritual gain. Nothing is allowed to happen in God's universe that can ultimately defeat His purposes. God is almighty, and who is mere man to say that God is not almighty? The Apostle Paul declared God's works all things that happen in life to His ultimate purpose. "We know that all things work together for good to those who love God." Romans 8:28 We need not worry about the future, because the Lord goes before us to prepare the way.

A vital part of the healing ministry is helping people face the fact of death and to receive the healing of their fears concerning their death. Many people have never thought of or felt through their dying. The value of a life is not calculated by its length of years but the quality of those years whether few or many.

What is the significance of the "will to live"? What is the meaning of being healthy? To what end are we to use our health? Do we use it to serve God, others, and ourselves? Yes! As the Westminster Confession of Faith affirms in its first question: What is the chief end of man? The chief end of man is to glorify God and to enjoy Him forever."

The realities of life and death are both good and evil. By our response to sickness we use it for greater service or we engage in self-pity. We have the freedom to make the choice. Illness, accidents and human tragedies can destroy our faith in God or enhance our faith in the positive response to these challenges. If the death and suffering of someone we love makes us bitter, jealous, against all religion, and incapable of happiness, we turn the person who died into one of the "devil's martyrs."

In contrast, if the suffering and death of someone close to us results in our giving more of our love in helping others, then we discover consolation and inner strength we never knew before. Several of the members of our cancer group have invested whatever life they have left by volunteering at the hospital to help others. They now experience a joy that they never knew before and a health they have not known for years. A common way of expressing it is that if life hands you a lemon, make lemonade out of it.

Many of the biological markers of aging are not valid at all. Rather they are markers of inactivity and poor nutrition. Investing your life in the lives of others keeps you feeling and looking younger. You get a "faith life" instead of a "face lift." Exercise is another key to youthfulness of body and spirit. Without exercise we grow old quicker and lose our childlike enthusiasm and joy.

CHAPTER 3

How Do We Know That God Heals?

We know through the testimony of the Bible. "Bless the Lord, O my soul, and forget not all his benefits: Who forgives all your sins and Who heals all your diseases." Psalm 103:2-3 God heals us now or at the time of our death when we receive a new body. Jesus said to her: "Daughter, your faith has made you well. Go in peace and be healed of your affliction." Mark 5:34 The Apostle reminds us that even faith is a gift from God. "And Peter said to Aeneas, 'Aeneas, Jesus the Christ heals you.'" Acts 9:34

Jesus knew what was inside a person, and His attitude towards that person was one of compassion. He was able to respond freely and directly to their needs, because He knew that there were causes of sickness and suffering beyond their control. Nowhere in the Gospels is there any suggestion of Jesus asking a sick person what he had done wrong before healing him. Instead Jesus took direct action to meet the person's need. Even the healing of the Gentile child in Matthew 15:22-28 was given freely and without any strings attached. In Jesus' day Jews were not to have any dealings with Gentiles, but Jesus saw everyone as a child of God.

Jesus was aware of the reality of alien and evil "spirits" that can get possession of a person. He also knew that God can touch an individual and not only drive out an evil spirit but also put God's Spirit in its place. Luke 11:22-28 Jesus was deeply aware that sick people were up against forces and realities which they could not handle on their own. He provided the love and strength needed.

Jesus' one mission was to bring the power and healing of God's creative and loving Spirit to heal the moral, mental, and physical illnesses of the people. It was a matter of rescuing people from a situation in which they were unable to help themselves. Jesus gave them new strength to bring them out of the pits of brokenness and sins. Modern medicine has adopted the same non-judgmental attitude toward patients. The New Testament is very clear that Jesus' disciples were to continue the ministry of God's healing Spirit.

Jesus used many different actions to heal the sick. He called upon the faith of the person. He touched the sick person. Jesus uttered commands. His most common means of healing were speaking words and touching the sick person. Often the two methods were combined and sometimes He used them separately. The "touch" method in the later history of the church became known as the "laying on of hands." When Jesus was in His home town of Nazareth, He was hindered by the unbelief of the people; yet He cured a few by the laying on of hands. Mark 6:5 When Peter cut off the ear of the servant of the high priest, Jesus reached out and touched the servant's ear; he was healed immediately. Luke 22:51

There are three instances when Jesus used saliva as a healing agent. Saliva was very common in the healing rites. Jesus used it not so much as a direct healing agent but as a carrier of His personality and power. In the Gospel of Mark we read of a man who was deaf and unable to speak. Jesus put His finger into the man's ear and touched his tongue with saliva, and then Jesus spoke the word: "Ephphatha" which means "be opened." Mark 7: 32-34 Although the Bible doesn't say that Jesus used oil in healing, He probably did as it was a very common practice in those days. Mark says the disciples "cast out many devils and anointed many sick people with oil and cured them." Mark 6:13 I use oil with patients when they request that I do so.

CHAPTER 4

The Power to Heal

What is faith? Faith is trusting in God's goodness in spite of what life events may bring. Faith is trust that God is at work in the adversities of one's life to bring about good for the person. Faith is also opening up the channels of our life to the healing power of God. Jesus' healings were part of His mission to bring people into a faith relationship with God.

The solution of every problem is to discover our peace in God, to see our oneness with divine reality, and to realize that we belong to God's family. We are here to be beneficial presences for others. Jesus' greatest work is the Crucifixion which for one thing shows that you cannot destroy God. The aim of life is to wake up completely and to see the hand of God working to make all things new. What blesses one blesses all.

Countless heroic souls have demonstrated the superiority of the spirit over the infirmities of the body. The late Christopher Reeves was a prime example of one who overcame his extreme handicap through faith in God. A man can overcome a disabling handicap, such as being a paraplegic, by finding the power to overcome it through faith in God. For Dr. Bernie Siegel the patient's life comes first; the disease is simply one aspect of his life. By a positive faith he can redirect his life in positive ways. Jesus knew the importance of a healed life, and He knew that a cure is often a by-product of healing. Jesus healed and cured through forgiveness and faith.

You may be wondering: "How is being a chaplain different from being a pastor? In the hospital the chaplain is in a different context and environment. Instead of chancels, pulpits, and congregations, the chaplain's ministry is at the bedside of a patient. The chaplain represents the spiritual concerns of the hospital towards the patient. The one-on-one situation provides a variety of opportunities to serve the patient different ways. The type of ministry is always initiated by the patient or by the patient's family or by one of the members of the hospital staff. The chaplain has the privilege of meeting many people each day and is honored to serve on the hospital team.

When I was serving as chaplain at Hollywood Presbyterian Medical Center in Hollywood, California, I visited a young female patient whose face was swollen with black and blue injuries to her eyes and her face. I asked her if she had been in an automobile accident. She said that her pimp had beaten her. Then she asked me if I knew of a place for helping prostitutes to get out of prostitution. I told her I would find out for her. I learned that there was a place in San Francisco led by a Christian group to help such women. She said she was very interested. So I called them, and they instructed me to put her on a bus, and they would meet her at the bus station in San Francisco. On day of her discharge I bought her a ticket and said goodbye to her as she boarded the bus.

About a year later I was waiting at the elevator at the hospital when a beautiful lady came up to me and said, "Chaplain Stover, I've been looking for you to thank you for your help." She could tell that I did not recognize her, so she told me that she was Debbie the former prostitute. I said, "Debbie, you look beautiful! What has happened?" She told me that she had met many men in her life, but at the Recovery Center she met a man that changed her life and she exclaimed, "His name is Jesus!" I rejoiced with her. What a wonderful story she has to tell as one whose life was changed through faith in the Lord's love and forgiveness!

Faith is the capacity of the soul to trust God and others. We can also express that faith in God as we place our trust in God's servants: doctors, nurses, and hospital staff. The challenge to our faith comes in our suffering. Suffering is at its root a moral issue which deals with values, priorities, and meanings. To listen to the voices of suffering in a hospital is a privilege which is given to a chaplain. Suffering dispels the illusion that we are indestructible and are without limits in what we can do. It is a moment of truth for most patients. Suffering can be redemptive and start us on the road of becoming well again.

One of the roles of the chaplain is to help patients face mortality, limits, priorities, and values. A supervisory nurse confidentially told me that she needed spiritual guidance. In addition to her job at the hospital she was the mother of several children; the wife of a wonderful husband and a student at a local college working on an advanced degree. Her schedule was so overwhelming that she didn't know how long she could handle all her commitments. She agreed with me when I said she needed to set some priorities. I asked her what she thought they were. She replied: my family first, my job, second, and my higher degree last. I agreed with her, and I inquired if she would like for me to pray for her, and she said, "Yes". After the prayer she said she felt much better and appreciated my confirmation of her priorities.

Several years ago I performed the wedding of a heart patient in his hospital room. My first question to him was: "Are you at peace with God?" I felt there was no time to delay the question since his doctor gave him a dire prediction of his impending death. He said that he was at peace with God and wanted to get married before he died. Some nurses served as witnesses, and we all had a joyful time during and after the wedding ceremony.

Another concern during times of suffering is one's productivity. The patient raises questions within himself: Who am I now? What can I still do? How can I express my love to my mate? What can I eat? Will my family and friends stand by me? How much longer will I have to see the doctor so often?

In the case of a cancer patient hope is often on a different level. She hopes she will be able to get through the radiation and chemotherapy without getting dreadfully sick. So many patients tell me that they smoked a lot and now regret having done so. I try to reassure them that God understands and will work to get them well under the circumstances. Or a patient will reveal their fear of a painful death more so than the fear of death itself. Sometimes denial of the disease shows itself in their doubt of the CT scan results.

Here are some of the ends of life issues: a Living Will, guardianship of their children, unfinished personal business, meaning of life, continuing care when they are discharged to home, and arrangements for a memorial service. "Two out of three deaths are premature." This statistic shows why doctors and medical people are dedicated to prolonging life for each patient. When Naaman the king was commanded by Elisha the prophet and king replied: "Are not the Abana and Pharpar, rivers of Damascus, better than all the waters of Israel? 2 Kings 5:12 The meaning of the "seven baths of the Jordan River 39 are:

1. The first bath is the washing of the outer skin. As a chaplain who visits patients I wash my hands many times especially if I touch the patient. Most hospital-related diseases result from staff and visitors forgetting or refusing to wash their hands.

2. Washing the inner skin. All of us are urged to drink no less than eight glasses of water each day to stay adequately hydrated. We need water to flush out our kidney and digestive system.

3. Cleansing the blood vessels. Exercise will accomplish this type of cleansing like stretching, walking, and resistance training.

4. Cleansing the lungs. Get outdoors for fresh air at least one hour a day.

5. Washing the emotions. Sigmund Freud was pestered by a persistent loquacious woman with an incurable disease. She insisted on coming to him and relating all her troubles. He frankly told her that the disease was incurable and that further consultation would be a waste of time for him and a waste of money for her. She said it was worth the cost to have the opportunity to share what was on her mind. Thus it was that psychiatry stumbled upon a method of healing that has revolutionized medicine. To drain out the poison from the emotions is as important as to drain out the poison from the body.

6. Washing the mind. An active, balanced and disciplined mind is one of the greatest sources of health a person can have. People who do not keep learning new things and keep their minds active get sick. "As a man thinks in his heart, so he is." Proverbs 23:7

7. Washing the soul. Many people are sick and burdened with guilt. Confession and forgiveness of sins is the way

to a cleansed soul. The way for Naaman to get well was to wash in the Jordan River seven times and to follow the directions given to him. In the classic, <u>The Pilgrim's Progress</u> by John Bunyan, Christian has a burden on his back that gets more difficult to bear. In spite of the burden Christian runs until he comes to a place somewhat ascending, and upon that place stood a Cross, and a little below in the bottom, a Sepulchre. Pilgrim in his dream sees that just as Christian came upon the Cross, his burden loosed from his shoulders, fell from off his back, and began to tumble until it came to the mouth of the Sepulchre where it fell into it, and he didn't see the burden anymore. I love this symbol of the effect of forgiveness of the burden of sin. When God forgives you, He lifts sin's burden, and the guilt vanishes from your life. You see it no more! We call this turning to God repentance.

Dr. Dean Ornish, known for his regimen for reversing heart disease says that the real health epidemic is spiritual heart disease. He defines it as loneliness and isolation. A doctor's caring regard for his patient will help the patient get well. The chronic diseases today are heart, cancer, diabetes, and obesity which are helped by love. Dr. Ornish says others made him feel special, and that caused him to feel loved.

Love by whatever method you discover it produces a new outlook, a new set of values, rebirth, and a new way of life. In its dramatic and instantaneous form we have the genuine conversion experience, always accompanied by some degree of healing whether physical, moral, mental, or emotional.

A woman saw engraved on the cornerstone of a fashionable church the instructions Jesus gave to His followers: "Heal the sick, cleanse lepers, raise the dead, cast out devils." Matthew 10 On impulse she walked around to the rectory door and asked to see the rector.

"I saw your sign," she said. "Do you?"

"Sign?" asked the bewildered rector, "Do I?"

"Do you 'heal the sick, cleanse the lepers, raise the dead, cast out devils'? If you don't, you shouldn't advertise it." Yes the church needs to practice what it preaches!

Does it matter to your body whether you live by God's principles and spirit or whether you live by the principles of our secular society? Or do you just do as you please? Either way your body reacts with health or sickness. The British Medical Association reports that there is not a single cell of the body totally removed from the influence of your mind and emotions.

How much do we place our trust in nutrition to cause our cells to function properly? "The Dietary Approaches to Stop Hypertension" study was a bold National Heart, Lung, and Blood Institute trial conducted at top four academic centers. They compared three different diets: a typical fatty American diet, a diet rich in fruits and vegetables, and a combination diet rich in fruits, vegetables, and low-fat dairy foods. The results were surprising. Everyone on the DASH diet achieved better health through the lowering of their blood pressure. It was a high potassium and calcium diet."[15]

What about worry? God has a sure cure for worry. Let the scriptures speak for themselves: Rejoice in the Lord always; again I will say, rejoice." Philippians 4:4 Let me give a personal example. When I was a child, I was teased by other children about being tongue-tied. I was embarrassed and avoided speaking in public which made the problem worse. In my senior year of high school I was to give a book report, and I purposely stayed home pretending I was sick. What made the change to now after preparing a sermon and preaching every Sunday for 30 years? I went to college and took English classes in which I had to speak before the class. Then I became a naval officer during World War II and had to stand before men and give orders. After the Navy I went to seminary and took speech classes for three years. It was the best thing that happened to me. I didn't worry how my speaking was coming across to others. I was healed of my worry and embarrassment about my speaking.

Frequently our hospital receives prisoners from a nearby state prison. The prisoners' legs are often chained to the bed. In addition two large armed guards prevent the prisoner from escaping. Their connection with the outside world was the medical personnel and me. I am thinking that the guards are a parable of worry and doubt dwelling within us and preventing our freedom to live a fuller life. They appear to be foreboding and dwarf us. Our freedom is to be found in the faith

---

15 Jeff Victoroff-<u>Saving Your Brain</u>, (Bantam Books/Random House, Inc., 2002) page 210

given us by the great physician, Jesus our Lord. "If the Son makes you free, you shall be free indeed." John 8:36 The Apostle Paul makes the same declaration, "Christ has made us free." Galatians 5:1

One of the greatest advances in modern medicine is the new vision that doctors are receiving in regards to the amount of control that a person may exert over the mental processes that influence the physical processes of the body. The results of countless placebo studies and the increasing use of biofeedback have caused medicine to undergo radical changes. It is no longer possible to see the body as a physical object waiting for replacement parts from the factory. Instead we now view the mind and body as an integrated system. What affects one affects the other.

In this view, physical treatment remains an integral part of the battle with a life threatening illness. Without considering the impact of the mind and spirit upon the patient the physical treatment is incomplete. Recovery is more likely to end with a positive result when we mobilize the whole person in the regaining of his health. The concept of the whole person requires that the patient plays an important role in regaining his health. The patient must do more than getting himself to the doctor so that the doctor can "fix" his ailing part.

A physician once said to me, "Patients want me to give them a magic pill without changing their lifestyle." Each person needs to assume responsibility for changing unhealthy attitudes and habits that do not move him or her in the direction of health. Stress may accumulate to the point where the individual can no longer cope with life and then becomes ill. When life becomes too hectic and when coping attempts fail, illness is the unhappy result. One of the leaders of our cancer group puts the blame of her cancer to the stressful relationships between her and her former husband. He left her with their two small children and married another woman with whom he had been having an affair. Stress does change the hormonal balance within the body which can compromise the immune system and prevent it from adequately defending the body against its internal enemies.

For most of human existence the demands placed on the nervous system were very different from those today. Our parents never heard of multitasking. Employees today are expected to be able to multitask. Stresses at work have greatly increased since our parents' day. Survival in primitive societies required the individual to be capable of immediately identifying a threat and making a quick decision whether to fight or flee. Life in today's society requires that we must frequently inhibit our fight or flight response. The body is designed so that moments of stress followed by a physical reaction such as fighting or fleeing do little harm. However, when the physiological response is missing, then the stress affects the body in a negative way.

Consider one critical area of life: marriage. Research confirms that faithfulness in marriage leads to a stronger immune system in which the white cells are strengthened to fight off infections. We were made to be true to our spouse, and when we are not, we are setting ourselves up for illness. That's why we promise to each other in the marriage ceremony that we will love each other "in sickness and in health and for richer or poorer until death does us part."

Evidence shows that stress predisposes people to illness. The time line is that illness follows a period of extreme stress within six to eighteen months of the stressful period. Our brain records feelings of depression and despair that are expressed in the limbic system in the form of illness. The limbic system is a series of pathways incorporating various structures deep inside the brain. A small area in the brain called the hypothalamus is the major way by which the limbic system affects the body.

The hypothalamus also affects the pituitary gland which in turn regulates the rest of the endocrine system with its vast range of hormonal control functions throughout the body. The net result of stress is that the immune system loses its ability to fight off invading infections. The same pathways are used to restore health. Sick patients need help in dealing with the stresses of their life. Hospital workers include social workers, finance counselors, chaplains, and other specialists. It is necessary to address all aspects of our illness in order to get well.

What are the spiritual conditions necessary for healing? The list would include a forgiving attitude and faith in God's goodness and His power to heal, patience for waiting upon God and His time frame of healing, love for God, others and yourself and staying in touch with God, one's own feelings and making the unconscious conscious through the help of a psychologist.

In the story of the paralyzed man brought to Jesus by his friends, Jesus said to him, "My child, your sins are forgiven." Mark 2:5 After another man had been healed Jesus saw him later in the Temple and told him, "Now that you are well again, be sure not to sin again or something worse may happen to you." John 5:14

Forgiveness of sins is the first step in reconnecting with God. Developing a positive attitude towards life when one is forgiven renews your spirit. You will not become perfect, so it is important to accept what you cannot change both in the past and in the present. Realize you cannot change others. Accept them as they are. With God's help you can change yourself-your attitude, your personality, and your habits –all by the grace and power of God.

Make the wonderful discovery of what you can be. God promises that you can live a worthy life through His love for you. "There's nothing more healing than to accept God's love." To know that you are loved by God so much that He gave His Son to die on a cross so that you are not only forgiven, but you are now a child of God. You belong to God, and you are a part of His royal family. Remind yourself that I'm really a wonderful person when Christ lives in me. "I can do all things through Christ who strengthens me." Phil. 4:13 There's no greater thing than to be used by God to continue the healing ministry of our Lord in whatever our calling may be in life.

Remember that you can handle all sickness through faith in your body's ability to heal you, in your doctor who is God's servant of healing, and in yourself as a complete person. The steps to mental, physical, and spiritual health are: patience, a trust in God's love, inspiration through the study of God's Words, prayer, enthusiasm, faith that acts, envisioning good results, and caring for others. Jesus said that even a faith as small as a mustard seed will produce amazing results in your life.

Many people criticize persons who believe that a positive faith can produce marvelous results. Positive thinking is also realistic thinking. It sees the negatives but it doesn't dwell on them. We have known many people who had a positive faith but died. That's right! Death is a part of every life, and positive thinking doesn't destroy that reality. But what was the quality of their dying and death? Did they live and die courageously, gallantly, and went into eternity with the glory that came from God? "Positive thinking cannot spare us from death, but positive thinking can help us die like great souls returning to our eternal home."[16] As a chaplain, I have seen how essential it is to have a positive faith to live each moment to the fullest.

---

16   Dale E. Galloway – Develop A Positive Attitude, (Tyndale House Publishers, Inc./ Wheaton, IL-1975) page 18

In getting and staying well, medicine alone cannot complete the job. Sick souls produce sick bodies. What we also need in our treatment plans is Christogenesis which means that everything that is whole begins with Christ. What can you do to make your world different? Get yourself full of the transforming power of God as revealed in Jesus our Lord that you become a dynamic and positive influence helping others to become well. "Surely goodness and mercy shall follow me all the days of my life, and I will dwell in the house of the Lord forever." Psalm 23:6 The essence of Christianity is newness. "Behold, I make all things new." Revelation 5:21 "If anyone is in Christ, he is a new creature. All things become new." 2 Corinthians 5:17

In Michelangelo's magnificent painting, The Creation of Adam, on the ceiling of the Vatican's Sistine Chapel, the extended right hand of God is reaching toward the outstretched left hand of Adam, but their hands do not touch. There remains the smallest of space between them. How can God and man connect with each other? It was the Cross of Jesus Christ that made the connection. Maybe Michelangelo believed that the gap needed to be filled by Divine action.

Christians often tend to be more perfectionistic than non-Christians. Many Christians are conscientious and have a desire to walk with the Lord, so they may worry a little more. Furthermore, because they have a fallen nature, they may have a tendency not to want to look at the truth about hidden emotions that are inconsistent with Scripture. The resulting internal conflict produces anxiety.

In the Old Testament an important word for anxiety is "kera", an Aramaic term, which describes a state of distress. Daniel used it to describe his distressed spirit. Daniel 7:15 Another Old Testament word is "charadah" which is used positively of the protective care the Shunammite woman for Elisha 2 Kings 4:13 A third term, "darash", is used of God's watchful and attentive care over the Promised Land and its Israelite inhabitants. Deuteronomy 11:12 Finally the Old Testament word is "daag" which means "to be afraid, careful." Sometimes "daag" carried the meaning of fear. The major word for anxiety in the New Testament is "merimma". The word comes from the idea of a distraction. "Merimma" can be positive in the sense of being careful or negative in the sense of overly anxious, distracted or distraught. Appropriate anxiety involves choosing to be distracted from self and to be focused on the needs of others. Inappropriate anxiety often produces stunted spiritual growth and leads to unfruitfulness. Anxiety involves forgetting God's personal care for us in all things.

One major technique in dealing with anxiety is a vital prayer life in which we have fellowship with God. Such prayer includes taking all our specific needs and concerns for others to God rather than trying to figure out what we can do about them. It is possible for a person who handles anxiety through prayer to experience worry-free living.

Fear is another hindrance for obtaining health. It is primarily a response to a threatening power by wanting to flee from it. In contrast to anxiety, fear has a specific object. Fear is also an appropriate response to spiritual danger. It is appropriate to fear engaging in a life style that you know is destructive to you physically and spiritually. The general attitude of the Christian is not to have a "spirit of fear". Fear of circumstances and adversities and the spirit of timidity or giving up on life are not to be marks of the Christian. One's health is a matter of being fully and dynamically connected to God.

CHAPTER 5

What Role Does Faith Play in the Healing Process?

Faith or trust in the physician's skill is necessary for the successful outcome of any treatment. One of the gospel writers is Luke who is identified as a physician-"Luke the beloved physician greets you." Colossians 4:14 In our cancer support group the members talked much about their doctors in complimentary ways. Sometimes they make unfavorable remarks. For instance, the group is opposed to the doctor telling his patient that he has only a definite time to live. They repeatedly say that the doctor isn't God. They agree that only God knows how long we will live. If the doctor gives them a time by which they will live, the patients believe their doctor and are likely to fulfill the doctor's expectations.

Physicians exert a powerful effect on their patients that affect the outcome of the treatment. If they strongly favor a certain kind of treatment, they can "talk it up" to the patient. My orthopedic surgeon strongly recommended that I have my aching knees replaced. I made an immediate date to have the surgery. I believed him, and both surgeries turned out well. It was confidence in his knowledge and skill that led me to have the knees replaced. The beliefs of the patient and the doctor ideally should coincide; and that is the best possible situation.

I shared with my primary doctor my award of a doctor's degree in theology. He said that my faith in God and in myself made it possible for getting the degree and began calling me Doctor Stover. He said, "You're a living example of the truth of your thesis." My thesis is : "The

Relationship Of Faith in God and Health." It made our relationship even stronger.

On the other hand, some doctors remain aloof from their patients. They believe in being objective all the time. Often they defend their detachment as one of the burdens of their profession. It is common for doctors to paint the worst possible outcome, and if things turn out better than predicted, the doctor is a hero. The custom of giving the cold facts to patients following diagnosis is prevalent. Patients who hear such comments as "You have a 25 percent chance of surviving this cancer" frequently interpret them to mean that I have a 75 percent of dying. It is to the patient's benefit to learn the doctor's way of relating to his patients.

The goal of a doctor ought never to obstruct the healing process by being unnecessarily pessimistic. Pythagoras, the ancient Greek mathematician, said that "the most divine art was that of healing. And if the healing art is most divine, it must occupy itself with the soul as well as with the body; for no creature can be sound so long as the higher part in it is sickly."

The greater one's faith in the medicine he is taking the more apt the medicine is to heal. Faith is the same whether we place it in a doctor or in God. The difference does not lie in the quality of the faith but the object to which the faith is directed. Religious faith is trust which the scientist puts in nature but is also extended to the sphere of the unseen where it becomes trust in the goodness of God. There is no tonic so uplifting and renewing as joy which sets into active exercise every constructive power of the body.

Even as late as the time of St. Augustine we find the belief in the healing power of faith still existing. In his City of God he describes various healing wonders of which he was an eyewitness and which were done in the name of Christ. Even if you have prayed for the preservation of the life of a loved one and that prayer was not answered in the way you had hoped, it is now hoped that you have reached the joyful conviction that your loved one is safe with God and that you will see him or her again.

Professor William James said, "As regards to prayers for the sick, if any medical fact can be considered to stand firm, it is that in certain environments prayer may contribute to recovery and should be encouraged as a therapeutic measure."[17]

---

17   William James-Varieties Of Religious Experience, (Random House/New York-1902) page 474

Dr. Charles Knuth, M. D., said that he now sees the spiritual dimension as integral to the practice of medicine, and I continue to work on helping clinicians incorporate the spiritual into patient contacts. The genius of Christianity is its fidelity to the permanent needs of human nature. In his book, Conquering Disability, Dr. Edgar Jackson writes that what a tragedy it would have been if I had not had the revelations that came with my stroke. We need help in finding positive aspects to the most negative happenings in life. We also need to be more understanding of those who are afflicted so that we may be as helpful to them as possible.

Life as we live it is a structure of relationships. One of the clearest indications of psychic injury is the loss of the sense of relationship. One of the adjustments to be made in the recovery from any kind of ailment is adapting to a new way of life. The process of recovery from a stroke is selective in nature. Healing is not quick or immediate but requires a long time. After my second knee replacement my surgeon said that he didn't want to hear any complaints until a year had passed. He was right in that I had no complaints even after eight months. In dealing with muscles of the body there is no substitute for careful training and dedicated effort.

A religious motive must exist to give meaning and purpose to life. Doubt cannot create that meaning. In times of crises to doubt the meaning of life is equivalent to disbelief. Illness and death are lost in a meaning larger than mere incidents in life. When we realize there must be a larger meaning to our existence, the process of living is no longer futile.

William James, Harvard professor who was quoted above, once said that pessimism is a religious disease. Why? It centers the focus on the self, making life increasingly selfish. In that kind of thinking all that comes into life is for the self. Where there is no outlet, as in the Dead Sea, bitterness develops. Any illness that focuses totally on the self ends in despair. The Christian faces life with a robust optimism that knows the worst and still believes in the best. It sees the darkness, the injustice and the sufferings of life, but it does not stop there. Christian faith goes beyond it knowing that its essence is selflessness. It finds in suffering the paradoxical truth that the self can be stronger than any of the things that come to it.

It is always a matter of choice based on a religious faith. Religion makes a venture of faith and finds a creative answer. Your recovery will be a time of triumph for body, mind, and spirit. It takes courage and faith to meet the struggles of life without giving up. It is important to know that our inner spirit is the primary resource for getting well again.

At the age of eighty-seven, Dr. E. Stanley Jones, the great missionary to India, suffered a paralyzing stroke. He wrote: "Now I must apply what I have preaching through the years: that no matter what happens to us, the final result depends on how we take it."[18] In the fourteen months following his book, The Divine Yes, Dr. Jones suffered a severe stroke. It is the story of his personal and triumphant spiritual victory when he said "Yes" to God and to his new life.

The Cross is the center of the Christian faith. God chose to use that defeat not to save Jesus but to save others through Jesus by that very suffering and death. God overcomes evil with good, hate by love and the world by a Cross through suffering. When one's life goes to pieces, take the pieces and give them to God. He will create a beautiful mosaic out of the pieces. It is amazing what God can do with a broken life when you give Him the pieces. When God puts the pieces together in a new form, we come to learn what wholeness and health really are. Jesus did not ask for a miracle of deliverance. He asked for the strength to drink the cup of bitterness and to endure the cross that He might pay the price of our redemption so that we could become whole in body, mind, and spirit.

The term "faith healing" is used uncritically about many non-physical ways of combating illness. There is healing through faith. Christian faith is the response of the whole man: thoughts, emotions, and will to the impact of God in Christ by which a person comes into a conscious, personal relationship with God. One can have healing without faith in Christ and have faith in Christ without healing. The Christian believes that God's ideal will is for us to have perfect health of body, mind, and spirit and to use every means of medical science, psychology, and every other relevant branch of knowledge to fight his way back to health.

Faith is enormously strengthened when Jesus is the object of faith, and when healthy emotions like love, trust, and admiration are expressed. What is done for the sick person is done by Christ who works through the patient's trust in Him. Faith means following the Lord whether healing comes or not. To yield one's life to God whether healing results or not is far more worthy of the name "faith" than the joy that comes only when

---

18   E. Stanley Jones-The Divine Yes, (Abingdon Press/New York-1975) page 33

one is healed. Sickness is more a mal-adjustment of the soul to God than the mal-adjustment of the body to the physical environment. Again God can use our suffering by weaving it into a pattern of his purpose in a manner that is beautiful and wonderful beyond our fondest dreams.

"I have affirmed the belief that the mind and one's attitude can make the body sick. But the opposite is also true: the mind and one's attitude can make the body well. Longevity is also affected by a happy marriage, plenty of rest, a strong faith in God, regular exercise, a well-planned diet, satisfying work, and relaxing play."[19]

My Aunt Carrie was born blind in the latter part of the 19th century. Every Sunday evening my mother would take me as a child to my grandmother's house where my Aunt Carrie lived. I use to wonder why she would sit in the next room in complete darkness listening to the radio while the rest of us sat in the kitchen. Years later I realized that Aunt Carrie's world was always dark, and it didn't make any difference where she sat. In those days there was little help for blind people.

Today causes of blindness in infants have been virtually eliminated with modern medicine and prenatal care. Though blindness is still an extraordinary burden to bear, the burden is made lighter by wonderful innovations. Books in Braille, guide dogs, and sound tapes are available. Blind students can attend and graduate from college with the help of computers that talk and tapes of lectures. Unfortunately, 73% of blind people are still unemployed.

We are always deciding what we will become in the next minute. Even retirement is not a tensionless state although many dream of that. The tension is between what one has accomplished and what goals one still needs to accomplish. It is healthier to be involved with life until the moment of death. The most challenging problem of human existence is suffering, and so I choose to be active in my retirement as a chaplain in four hospitals. I want to be there for people who are suffering.

"To live is to suffer; to survive is to find meaning in the suffering. The feeling needs to be awakened in us that we are responsible to life for something, however grim our circumstances may be. There is only one thing I dread and that is not to be worthy of my sufferings." Dr. Frankl learned that caring for the other prisoners and sharing what little he had to share was the attitude that saved his life. He made the life-changing and life-saving decision to live for the other prisoners.

---

19   Robert A. Schuller-The World's Greatest Comebacks, (Harper/San Francisco-2000) page 128

Faith in the healing processes of your body is required to keep your health. "Do you not know that your body is the temple of the Holy Spirit who is in you, whom you have from God and you are not your own?" I Corinthians 6:19 We are not only responsible to others and our self for taking good care of our body but also to God who wants to use our body for His good purposes. Jesus brings out the resources of God's Kingdom that reside within us. The Westminster Confession of Faith declares in its opening question: "What is the chief end of man? The chief end of man is to glorify God and to enjoy Him forever." Dr. Albert Schweitzer who gave up a prosperous opportunity as a surgeon to help the people of Africa said that in the hands of the Master, we become diamonds who sparkle with the love of God. Whenever he played his worn-out piano, it produced heavenly music.

Nothing is more remarkable about the human body than its recuperative powers. Hippocrates, the first major name in medicine, was both a theoretician and a practitioner. He tried to close the gap between the understanding of disease and its treatment. He was holistic in his approach to disease when he insisted that it is natural for the human body to heal itself even without the intervention of a physician. He believed that the essential function of the physician was to avoid any treatment that might interfere with the natural healing processes. He gave the admonition which every physician learned early in training and practice: "Do no harm."

What is important in recovering one's health is not the laying on of tools but the laying on hands. When the patient hears his doctor say, "Yes, you have had a heart attack, but you are going to recover." Many people allow illness to disfigure their lives more than it should. They give up needlessly, not realizing the powers within their bodies for healing. There is always a margin in which life can be lived with meaning and even with a certain measure of joy.

However, victory over a disease often comes through a paradox. Alcoholics are advised that victory comes through surrender. A paradox is a statement or experience that appears to be contradictory. Paradox was not foreign to Jesus. He taught: "He who finds his life will lose it, and he who loses his life will find it." Matthew 26:25 Embracing such opposite views Jesus was pointing to a larger truth.

We are a paradox. We were created "living beings" out of dust and clay. Like the beasts of the fields we share common drives. We are bounded by time and will die. Yet that doesn't fully describe us. We are fashioned "in the likeness of God–in God's image." This term is used exclusively in the book of Genesis. The similarity or likeness is not a physical one but a similarity of powers and capacities not shared to the same degree by other creatures. Like God, we are self-aware and self-transcendent. We can know and relate to our Creator God because of the manner in which He made us.

Are we caring for our bodies like we should? The Surgeon General of the United States reported that fifty-five percent of Americans are significantly overweight and sixty-two percent do not exercise. The abundant life which Jesus promises begins with learning to take care of ourselves in healthy ways.

I have made an acronym that reminds us of the things we need to do to be healthy: W.A.D.E. S. It stands for Weight, Attitudes, Diet, Exercise, and Spirituality. All five components of the acronym contribute to a sound body for the Spirit of God to inhabit. Jesus by His very nature brought life and healing to people He met. He also showed that His power was greater than the power of the Evil one when Jesus cast out demons. He defeated the power of evil on the Cross and ultimately in His Resurrection.

Through the complex medium of His own compassion and the sick person's faith, the healing became a sacrament of God's love and power. It is interesting that Jesus could not perform any great acts of healing in His hometown of Nazareth because of their disbelief. People perceived Him as another carpenter in their village. The proverb explains it all: "A prophet is not without honor except in his own hometown."

The most significant reason Jesus healed was that He had compassion on people and suffered when they did. The root meaning of compassion is: "suffering with." Jesus opposed sickness, because it caused needless suffering. In cultures where the spirit of Christ is not known, this compassion is often conspicuously lacking.

I recall an incident in the hospital when I was called to the bedside of a patient who just died. The wife was a Buddhist. She was crying and apologized to me for her tears. She said that her faith teaches her not to cry. I stayed with her until the Buddhist monk arrived. I experienced aloofness from the monk towards the wife. He did not touch her nor shed any tears. Jesus in contrast cried at the tomb of Lazarus and had compassion on the crowd because they were without a shepherd.

Modern medical practice is a monument to the spirit of Jesus who by His example taught that healing is a good work of God. It was like pulling an ox out of a pit--important and valuable enough to break the Sabbath law. Humans are of great worth and whatever contributes to their restoration and health is also of great value. Healing in and of itself is good.

When people came to Jesus in faith and humility, He healed them as a response to their trust in Him and out of His love for them. When a man asked Jesus to heal him, he exclaimed: "Lord, I believe; help the little faith that I have." Mark 9:24 Jesus healed in part to increase his faith. Healing is one way of opening the people's eyes to the wonderful nature and power of God. They may begin or renew their faith. Healing increases faith, and faith increases healing.

Jesus healed the sick to help them find the wholeness they desired. He was aware of the relationship between sin and sickness and of the need for a spur such as illness to move them toward wholeness. He showed the connection between sin and sickness in the healing of the invalid in John 5:14, "See, you have been made well. Sin no more, lest a worse thing come upon you." Jesus never made personal sin the sole or most important cause of sickness. People who have lost their way find themselves exposed to destructive spiritual forces that have often triggered emotional and physical disturbances. There is good medical evidence that such disturbances contribute to a variety of physical illnesses. There is clearly a very direct connection between sin and sickness.

The relationship between faith in a loving God and the healing of the body, mind, and spirit is a direct one. Love is the answer as revealed in Jesus' healing of the sick. Is death the final act when we shall receive a new body? God either takes away the disease from us, or He takes us away from the disease.

Many today are far too dependent upon pills and other means of healing. Millions are running from doctor to doctor gobbling down pills and taking all types of medicines. The proper balance between faith in the Lord and medicine will be better kept if we pursue the following:

1. Appreciate and believe that the Lord is the final healer regardless of the channel for healing.

2. Realize that medicine will never have the complete answer for the illnesses and problems of the human race.

3. Permit the Living Christ to rule your life and actions.

4. Do not become dependent upon the wonders of medicine.

5. Realize that spiritual healing is the prime goal. The wholeness of our spirit is the greater need.

6. Give thanks and praise to the Lord for your healing regardless of the method He used to make us well.

7. Minister with prayer to all who are in any way in need of healing. Faith in the Great Physician is expressed in prayer to the Lord. William James said that prayer is the very soul and essence of religion. He also said that there is no intimate conversation, no interior dialogue, no interchange, and no action of God without prayer. An individual has not done all he can about the healing of a disease until he has prayed.

When it comes to healing something radical takes place in consciousness. Not only do we begin to understand the meaning of our suffering but also the spiritual aspect of the illness. When that happens, something more takes place than a relief of the symptoms. We are able to see something and understand something that previously we did not. Ordinarily people feel sorry for themselves for having suffered, but in cases where complete healing takes place, there is a sense of gratitude for the experience. It brought a realization which is of great value to the individual. "Once we understand the true nature of healing, there is a valuable lesson in it for us all. If we have a problem, we may embrace it and say with Jacob when he wrestled with the angel: "I will not let you go until you bless me." Genesis 32:26

We live in a universe where the spirit is real and dynamic. Physicists tell us that what appears to be solid is really energy moving all the time. Even our bodies are mostly space. If you were to remove all the space between the molecules in the human body, a dot barely discernible to the human eye would be left. The walls of your rooms are nothing more than an electric field that resists penetration. Jesus passed through the door of the house where His disciples were hiding on the night of His Resurrection. We are really mainly spirit that uses the mind and the body to express itself in sickness or in health.

Dr. James Lynch, a medical researcher at John Hopkins Medical Center, affirmed his absolute conviction that loneliness is the number one killer in America today. When I make my rounds at the hospitals, I notice the presence or absence of flowers. Flowers are a sign that the patient is in a loving relationship with others who help make recovery a greater possibility. Patients who are members of a loving congregation will joyfully tell me that their pastor came to see them and to pray for them.

Cancer cells have a way of letting us know that we live by grace moment by moment. Cancer breaks our cells into many pieces and like a puzzle our body is challenged to put them together. Cancer takes away a part of you: a breast or a prostate or a kidney or a lung or a section of your colon. Treatment for cancer often takes away your hair and your bowel control. In spite of all that as one cancer patient said to me: "Cancer has brought me closer to God and to those who love me and to my real self."

The Bible reminds Christians that they are a fellowship of priests with the power to be a channel of healing for others. "You are a royal priesthood." 1 Peter 2:9 One can turn away from the ill person like a tribal community rejects a person who is hexed by the witch doctor. A few years ago, I was asked to give a prayer at the 100th birthday of a member of our church. It was a festive occasion with balloons and lots of food. The honored guest was invited to make any remarks about reaching the century mark. He got up and said: "This is the day the Lord has made. I will be glad and rejoice in it." Psalm 118:24 He shared with the celebrants that he repeated this verse every morning upon awakening through his entire adult life and concluded with thanks to everyone for coming to celebrate his birthday. His doctor was there to help celebrate this momentous occasion.

About a month later he telephoned me to come to see him. When I got there he said that his daughter had arranged for him to go to a residential home and leave his house the following day. He remarked to me, "I'd rather be dead than to move to a place like that!" He was so unhappy. What a contrast in his spirit compared to the day of his 100th birthday celebration! I prayed for him lifting up his burden to God. The next morning his daughter called me to tell me that her father had died during the night. He had gone to his Heavenly home to be with his wife and his Lord.

CHAPTER 6

The Healing Process

What happens to our body in the healing process? For one thing faith enables the brain to release endorphins and other chemicals that enhance the healing process. Faith in God stimulates the will to live and activates the healing properties within the body. The body has its own apothecary.

Let's begin with the brain which sets us apart from all other creatures. It is the organ by which we think and store memories which recall our personal history. It keeps all the other parts of the body functioning and is dependent upon the heart for its supply of nutrients to keep it healthy. The thoughts and emotions of the brain affect the health of the rest of the body. When the doctor pronounces the patient "brain dead", he means that there is no longer a medical possibility that the person will live.

The medical team (like mechanics) is primarily responsible for our body. However, we are responsible for taking good care of our body as long as we live. Greg Anderson, a cancer survivor, wrote in his book, <u>Cancer Conqueror</u>, "I knew that I had to rededicate myself to living that one day for all it was worth." We need to educate ourselves on any disease that may come to us because that is vital to our getting well. It's important to remember that you might have cancer, but you are not cancer. Separate your personhood from the disease. Who I am as a person is much more important than the disease I have for now.

Cancer cells are confused cells that don't know where they belong or when to stop dividing. Again, our immune system is the mortal enemy of cancer cells. All treatments aim at helping the immune system to stay strong in the fight for health. God's Word also reminds us who our greatest ally is: "He sent His word and healed them." Psalm 107:20

Cancer is not a disease of which you are a victim. It is a process which you can master with God's and medical help. Cancer is not primarily a noun but a verb. A cancer patient is going through a process called cancer. This shifts the focus from a disease to a process which can be reversed. Our genes, our environment, and our food can trigger the cancer process. The process can also be initiated by a prolonged emotional conflict that has its base in stress. The tumor is a signal to the body that we need to make some changes in our life.

Unless we have a healthy respect for ourselves, we probably won't eat a balanced diet, exercise, and stop smoking. The development of cancer requires more than just the presence of abnormal cells. It requires a suppression of the body's natural defenses. When we do not exercise, then the stress is internalized which sets up the body for illnesses of all kinds. We need to examine the emotions behind the stress that invariably have roots in fear, anger, or guilt.

The heart of the immune system is the person's white blood cells. Recently in an amazing discovery white blood cells were shown to have neuroreceptors. This means that our feelings and emotions can be biochemically transmitted to the immune system. You become a cancer conqueror not because you go into remission. Instead, you become a cancer conqueror because you choose to become a new person.

The new person realizes that the value of one's life is not in its duration but in its donations of love. Research was done on women having breast biopsies. The group that reacted best were those whose first action and attitude was prayer. Prayer has been shown to reduce stress hormones. Another way the stress hormones are reduced is involvement with helping others. The path to health is commitment to action that makes society and the environment healthy. "Man carries the world in his head," wrote Ralph Waldo Emerson, "the whole astronomy and chemistry suspended in a thought. Because the history of nature is carried in his brain, therefore he is the prophet and discoverer of her secrets."

We are greater than the sum of our biological parts. We also have the capability to be better than we are at present. You're a lot better off if you just keep going. I've known plenty of people who've had cancer and some awful thing happened to them. They seem to do very well as long as they keep positive even if it doesn't give them any longer life. Giving up is a form of suicide. There are others who need us - whether our children or extended family. Each of us has a purpose on this earth.

Marcus Aurelius, considered wisest man of ancient Rome, said: "Our life is what our thoughts make of it." Even earlier Solomon wrote: "As a man thinks in his heart, so he is." Proverbs 23:7 Choosing to live joyfully makes a huge difference in getting well, because it affects the functioning of the immune system in a very positive way.

Norman Cousins, author of "An Anatomy Of An Illness" relates his story of success in regaining his health. His primary point is that the patient has most of the responsibility for recovery to health. He beat the odds that he would die soon after his heart attack by using the power of laughter, courage, and tenacity. He affirmed that positive emotions are powerful weapons in the war against illness. By his own life he demonstrated what the mind and the body working together can accomplish in overcoming illness. Norman encourages every patient to be a participant in his/her own treatment.

Dr. Carl Simonton investigated why some patients respond very well to treatment. In interviews he found a familiar theme: all had very strong reasons to get well: to see my daughter graduate from high school or be at my son's wedding or to hold my new grandchild yet to be born. All these got well because they had strong reasons to live.

Goals make life worth living. "For me to live is Christ." Philippians 1:21 For the Christian serving Him makes life worth living as we share His love with others. Faith in Him is a great resource for renewing one's health. When one is fighting a life-threatening disease, it takes courage to live and to engage in the struggle for health. Most people believe that if they were told that they had a life-threatening disease, they would do all the things they had put off doing and would live life to the hilt. Society calls this the "bucket list."

To have good health it is necessary to pay attention to one's needs- mental, physical and spiritual and then act to fulfill those needs. The most effective tool for taking specific positive action is to set new goals. For some this is the first time they have formulated their goals to accomplish in life. Living longer insists on your meeting your needs and setting goals. The will to live is stronger when there is something for which to live.

Other benefits from goal setting are:

1. Setting goals prepares you mentally and emotionally to act out your commitment to regain your health.

2. Setting goals expresses confidence in your ability to meet your needs. You are declaring that you are in charge of your life. You are acting upon life rather than life acting upon you. This self-assertive stance runs counter to the feelings of hopelessness and helplessness.

3. Setting goals builds a positive self-image.

4. Setting goals provides a focus for your energy which then stimulates your immune system

5. Setting goals establishes priorities and moves you in the direction you want to go.

6. Setting goals gets you involved in your daily living whether you achieve all your worthwhile objectives or not. It is the striving to meet your goals, not their ultimate fulfillment, that gives meaning to life. Goals can be changed as your priorities change. New ones can be added and others can be dropped.

What happens to the mind in healing? The mind opens to the avenues of God's power to cure. When one has faith that he will accomplish his goals, the projected outcome is more likely to happen.

Glenn Clark wrote in his book, How To Find Health Through Prayer, "I used to wonder why a rotten apple placed in a barrel of sound apples would not make all the rotten apples sound. I also wondered why a man infected with small pox when turned loose in a gathering of sound people would make many of them sick. I also wondered why a healthy person walking through a hospital would not make sick people well. In other words, I wondered why God had made a universe where soundness and health seemed futile and sickness seemed contagious.

But one day I stopped wondering and examined the so-called sound apple, and I found it was not sound. It was lacerated, torn and wounded to the death. Look beyond the apple to the stem. There in its most vital part of all you would find the mortal wound. You would find that the apple was torn away from its parent tree. It had been hopelessly separated from its source of life. When I discovered this, I learned one of the truest facts of life: that nothing, whether it be fruit or vegetable or man, when separated from its source is sound."[20]

The Bible's story of this separation is told in the Creation story. The disobedience of Adam and Eve separated them from God, and they were denied perfect existence in the Garden of life where God had originally placed them. That mortal wound of sin has been transmitted to all humans ever since. Connection with God is restored through the life, death, and resurrection of Jesus.

Dr. Caroline Thomas, a psychologist at John Hopkins University, interviewed more than 1300 students and followed their history of illness. The most distinctive profile belonged to students who developed cancer. Those students saw themselves as having experienced a lack of closeness with their parents. They seldom demonstrated strong emotions and were generally in low gear. They tended to be prone to feelings of hopelessness and helplessness even before the onset of cancer.

Many cancer patients have difficulty expressing their negative feelings and have the need to constantly look good to others. The major difference between heavy smokers who get lung cancer and heavy smokers who do not get cancer is that the lung cancer patients have "poorly developed outlets for emotional discharge." The difficulty for the patients with fast-growing tumors seemed to be that the emotional outlets were blocked by an extreme desire to make a good impression. When a person is emotionally trying to defend himself and always trying to look good, it requires so much energy that the patient doesn't have energy to fight the cancer.

Retiring from one's work can impact one's health. One executive in a large firm had always felt important. When people asked him what he did, he would answer that he was retired. He noticed he did not get the spark of interest and respect that he had been used to. He also missed the excitement of his work.

Dr. Lawrence Le Shan, an experimental psychologist by training and a clinical psychologist, is one of the foremost theorists of the psychological life history of cancer patients. In his book, You Can Fight For Your Life, he identifies four typical components in the life stories of more than 500 cancer patients with whom he worked. The patient's

---

20   Glenn Clark-How To Find Health Through Prayer, (Harper & Brothers Publishers/ NY – 1940) page 40

youth was marked with feelings of isolation, neglect, despair, and with intense interpersonal relationships appearing difficult and dangerous.

In early adulthood the patient was able to establish a strong and meaningful relationship with a person or to find great satisfaction in his vocation. A tremendous amount of energy was poured into this relationship or job. It became the reason for living and became the center of the patient's life. Then the center was removed through divorce, death, a move, a child leaving home, or retiring from the job. The result was despair as though the "bruise" left over from childhood had been painfully struck again. One of the fundamental characteristics of these patients was the despair that had been "bottled up." These individuals were unable to let other people know when they were hurting, angry and hostile. Others frequently viewed them as unusually wonderful people, saying of them, "She's such a good, sweet woman. She's a saint."

Dr. Le Shan concludes: "The benign quality, the 'goodness' of these people, was in fact a sign of their failure to believe in themselves sufficiently and their lack of hope." The growing despair that each of these people faced appears to be strongly connected with the loss that each suffered in childhood. They saw the end of the relationship as a disaster that they had always half expected. They had been waiting for it to end and waiting for rejection. When it happened, they said to themselves: "Yes, I know it was too good to be true." The color, the zest, and the meaning went out of their lives. They no longer seemed attached to life. It is better to stay in a shell. There they stayed waiting without hope for death to release them. Seventy percent of all the cancer patients Le Shan interviewed shared this basic emotional life history.

How can one counteract the stress on the body? Physical exercise is part of the answer. The Hebrew people in capturing Jericho got very involved physically by walking around the walls of the city once for six days and then on the seventh day, they walked around seven times. All of this physical activity helped them in handling the stress of battle. Jesus spent a lot of time walking in His three years of ministry. Prior to this He did carpentry work which is also physically demanding. To our knowledge Jesus was never sick.

When I was in Midshipmen's School, we worked very hard to get ready for our part in the war. I had to run up seven flights of stairs with my books or my military gear in addition to the calisthenics five times a week. Since then, I have trained for the Los Angeles Marathon which requires lots of training in addition to the challenge of the marathon. I can honestly say that the physical exercise relieved me of the stresses of being a chaplain. I learned from my navy experience that it is important to be in good physical condition to do any task to the best of my ability.

Bereavement also lowers the immune system and makes us more susceptible to illness. In the second century A. D. the physician Galen observed that cheerful women were less prone to cancer than women of a depressed spirit. I have led Grief Recovery groups for twenty years. It is wonderful to watch people express their emotions and the changes that result in their life since being in a support group.

One of my grief recovery members lost her daughter when one of her daughter's co-workers murdered her and stuffed her body in a large garbage container. When the mother came to the group, she was hysterical for weeks. She would repeat the awfulness of the murder with which we all agreed. By the time the last session came she had calmed down considerably and was even able to laugh when something funny was said by members of the group. She had begun to work through the emotional upheaval of such a tragedy.

If the patient believes he is not being treated with respect than that belief interferes with the healing. My experience is that the vast majority of nurses and hospital staff genuinely care for the patient and show great respect for them. It's critical to know what was going on in your life before you got sick. Were you getting enough sleep? What were some of the stresses happening in your life? Am I seeking some benefit from my illness? These are important questions.

What are the benefits of illness? It allows you to engage in behavior that you can't do when you are well. When ill, you can stay home and not go to work. You have neighbors who will attend to some of your chores. Neighbors and friends bring meals. You can order "meals on wheels." Sometimes such acts of kindness can be an obstacle to being normal. You can come to enjoy the attention and being waited on.

When Jesus met the man by the pool who had been sitting there for thirty-eight years, He asked him if he wanted to get well. He said that he did. Jesus then commanded him to take up his bed and walk. How amazing! When we are sick, people bring us flowers, send us cards and come to see us. We enjoy the increased attention and acts of kindness. Then when we are discharged, we have access to the best parking spots. Sickness does have its benefits. Most of us, however, prefer to be well and take care of ourselves.

Dr. Carl Jung, the psychiatrist, wrote: "The life of the body is the soul but the life of the soul is God."[21] When we are connected to God, we are whole and as the hymn says: "It is well with my soul." Dr. Jung discovered in exploring the depths of his patients' soul that the soul includes both the good and the evil within us. "Like the frog in the fairy tale was transformed into a handsome prince when the princess kissed the frog, so our inner enemy is changed into a useful part of our personality. It is not the enemy within who is evil; it is our unawareness of the enemy which creates evil. To achieve wholeness we must bring all the parts of our personality together, both the good and the evil. A healing part of the worship service is acknowledgement of our evil and finding forgiveness.

Most of us fear getting ill because it disrupts our life. We may become so incapacitated that someone else must wipe our bottom. The most personal and basic things are taken from us. When I had my last knee replacement, I remember the nurse coming in one morning and saying that she was going to give me a shower. Oh no! With the exception of breathing and eating we become dependent on others.

Mitch Albom writes: that I am an independent person, so my inclination was to fight all this--being helped from the car and having someone else dress me. I felt a little ashamed because our culture tells we should be able to wipe our own bottom. We enjoy God and others when we realize that their caring is an expression not only of their caring but also God's love.

"Man often has fear stamped upon him before his entrance into the outer world; he is reared in fear; all this life is past bondage to fear of disease and death; and thus his whole mentality becomes cramped, limited, and depressed, and his body follows its shrunken pattern and specification."

The Bible speaks of a key to victory in life. It talks about the key that inevitably leads to triumph: the key of faith. "Faith is the victory that overcomes the world." 1 John 5:4 By faith I mean a conscious decision to place my entire life under the care of God who loved me enough to die on the cross for me. When a person has major surgery, she trusts the surgeon even though she has no real understanding of how he is going to operate or what will be the final outcome of the surgery. She trusts him, and she understands that the surgeon's work will enable her to get well.

---

21 Wayne G. Rollins-Jung And The Bible, (John Knox Press/Atlanta-1983) page 126

St. Augustine said that God wants to give us something, but cannot, because our hands are full. One way God gets our attention is to allow us to experience pain. "Pain is unmasked, unmistakable evil. Everyone knows that something is wrong in our body when it hurts. Pain insists upon being attended to. God whispers to us in our pleasures, speaks to our conscience, and shouts to us in our pain."

Zach Thomas in his book, <u>Healing Touch</u>, shows how the Gospel calls for respectful, appropriate "heart, hand coordination" for the healing of the whole person. He experienced the healing touch himself which aroused his faith in God. This experience spurred him to travel to other cultures to learn how they give primary attention to massage and human touch in their healing arts. Jesus' ministry highlighted healing touch. Early Christians used healing touch in their homes and rituals. Somewhere along the way we lost it. We passed it on to clergy, then to medical professionals, and even to 'faith healers'. In so doing, we unwittingly forfeited a heartfelt way of expressing the Christian faith.

In the early church Christians expected physical cures to accompany the laying on of hands in baptism, communion, and special services for the sick just as the ancient Greeks left offerings to their healing god, Asclepius, in appreciation for recoveries they attributed to his "divine touch".

One day I received a call from the hospital to administer final spiritual ministrations to a twenty-year old female who was slipping rapidly into brain death. She was thrown through the windshield of her car as she had not worn her seat belt. I anointed her with holy oil on her forehead, making the sign of the cross with the oil; baptized her; shared scripture and prayed. I hugged her parents, grandparents, and her boyfriend. I touched each person present. They thanked me for what I had done for their daughter.

The central convictions of Christianity are being lost. The fault does not lie completely with the perversity and secularism of the culture in which we live. Sometimes the fault lies in the fact that people have not been given the opportunity to discover the healing power of Christ. Health is a combination of all that has happened to you.

"After eating the forbidden fruit Adam hid himself with his wife behind the trees in the garden. Then the Lord God called to Adam and said, "Adam! Where are you?" Genesis 3:9 At that point in the story pastoral care was born. Spiritual care attempts to discover the true situation of a person with whom it is concerned. Man must recognize that he is hiding, must see the trees which serve him as a hiding place, and, in the end, must understand the reasons that drove him to this dissimulation.

When Pilate presented Jesus to the howling mob, dressed up in ridiculous symbols of royalty, he unknowingly made a proclamation of infinitely greater import than he realized: "Behold the Man!" John 19:5 Behold the man, indeed! He is the sorrowful bearer of the sin which indwells and destroys humanity: behold the man!

At the same time Pilate shows us the Man: man such as he should be, the human type, man in every sense of the word, the man we all ought to be. He is the one, indeed, who fulfilled in himself my destiny. If I want to know who I am, if I want to know who I am called to be, I have only to look at Jesus. He shows all my possibilities and unveils for me the object of my human existence.

Man, true man as God wanted him to be, is only met in the person of the Son of Man, Jesus Christ. Apart from Christ we are not what we ought to be. We have not accomplished God's plan for us. In Jesus Christ God gives us the full vision of the man He had wanted from the beginning, the man we are called to become.

When we are prepared to see in Jesus the Christ, the perfect image of the existence which was intended for us, His life is the event whose importance we cannot adequately describe. Christian pastoral care aims at bringing a human being to faith in Christ so that he may accomplish his true destiny as man. Sickness is everything which hinders man in his path towards his full humanity. We see an example of this in Joni Eareckson's response to her disability. She discovered that God brought healing of her attitude of spirit and mind which enabled her to live a life of strong purpose in spite of her physical handicap.

That is why healing goes beyond the single task of restoring a physiological function. Jesus' work of healing unveils to us the will of the Most High to restore the reign of God to the whole of His creation, including the healed person.

CHAPTER 7

In What Way does the Church Continue the Healing Ministry of Jesus?

Jesus told His disciples to heal the sick. The Church is commissioned to carry on the work of healing. "I tell you most solemnly, whoever believes in Me will perform the same works as I do myself. Whatever you ask in My name I will do so that the Father may be glorified in the Son." John 14:12-14

The Church prays for the sick. What is the role of prayer in the healing ministry of the Church? Dr. Larry Dossey, author of <u>Healing Words</u>, wrote in an article that prayer is good medicine. He claims that praying for oneself and others makes a scientifically measurable difference in recovering from illness. In his article he tells us we can make the most of our own healing prayers. Dossey emphasizes that praying is not a replacement for medical treatment, but instead is a very effective addition to it.

The Church prays for the sick in the worship services. In our church we provide opportunity for the worshippers to write a request that is placed on the offering plate followed by the minister praying for each person so named. Then on Monday the requests are sent out to prayer partners via e-mail.

The word prayer derives from the Latin "precarious", obtained by begging and the word precari-to entreat-to ask earnestly. This suggests two of the most common forms of prayer: petition, asking something for one's self, and intercession, asking something for others. Prayer may be individual or communal. It may be offered in words, sighs, gestures, or silence. Prayer is often a conscious activity, but it may also flow from depths of the unconscious, as in dreams. A complete definition of prayer cannot be given because of its vastness and complexity.

For the Christian, spiritual healing is rooted in the love of God revealed in the work and teaching of Jesus. The early Church engaged in the spiritual healing ministry as a prominent part of the proclamation of the Gospel. Both the past and the present work of the Church's healing ministry are rooted in the Divine Commission to "heal the sick." Mathew 10:8

The Reverend Donald W. Bartow, pastor emeritus of the Westminster Presbyterian Church in Canton, Ohio, writes about the results from one of his prayer healing services. One man attended seeking help for his severe arthritis. He had been in constant pain which prevented him from working. During the healing service he experienced freedom from pain and from stiff joints. The next day he was able to return to work.

A woman at the same service who was also suffering from arthritis found no relief. She did testify that she was healed of a resentment that she had carried for many years. A visiting pastor who felt defeated was also at the service. He was planning to leave the pastorate because he could not get along with the members of his church for whatever reason. When he received the laying on of hands, he was set free from his anger. He realized the problem was not the members, but he was the problem. He decided to remain in his pastorate.

Prayer is a medical and scientific issue. Today over 130 controlled scientific studies investigating the effects of intercessory prayer have been carried out, and over half of these reveal statistical evidence that prayer has a significant effect on the person who prays. In addition, more than 250 studies show that, on average, religious practices that include prayer promote health. Prayer is universal. Plutarch, the ancient Greek biographer and historian, observed that if we traverse the world, it is possible to find cities without walls, without wealth, without schools, or theatres. No one has been able to find a city without a temple or worship place. People throughout the history of mankind have prayed because they needed the help of a higher power.

We have looked at the Gospel record, and it does make real spiritual impact affecting the body, emotion, and spirit. We need to remember how special Christian healing is as we know it in scriptures and throughout the world today. The Apostle Paul warned the Church at Corinth about punishing themselves with sickness for their misuse of the Lord's Supper. In addition to specific healings there are ten incidents of healing in the book of Acts which refer to the healing of large numbers of people by the Apostles. Acts 2:23 In Acts 5:15 it records that the sick were brought out on beds and couches into the street so that as Peter passed by his shadow might fall on them and make them well. A crowd from the cities around Jerusalem also came bringing their sick, and they were all healed.

One is struck by the quality of expectation on the part of sick when you read these stories. As Geddes Mac Gregor writes in his exposition on the book of Acts, "There can be no question that the first Christians lived in daily expectation of 'miracles' and may well have experienced them." Interpreter's Bible, volume 9:53. Pagans who were healed by the early Christians turned with joy and amazement to the church. Not all who were converted thanked Jesus. Neither did all the healed ten lepers return to thank Jesus for their healing except one. After all, if simple ordinary people have access to divine power, it is impressive. These men seemed to have a power and a spirit other than their own which worked through them to heal the sick.

The minister or priest walks into the sickroom as the duly ordained representative of Him who said, "For I was hungry, and you gave me food; I was thirsty, and you gave me drink; I was naked, and you clothed me; I was sick, and you visited me." Matthew 25:35-36 To be sick is to be a stranger among strangers. To be sick is to pass through strange places of the spirit: the night before an operation with its haunting dreads and imaginings, the taking of an anesthetic and the struggle with post-operative discomforts.

The power of God can be manifested in a person's life bringing about a cure of the illness or a triumph of the human spirit or both when it is aided by God. God's aid to strengthen the patient's faith comes through the ministry of Church's love and caring in the work of the pastor and the congregation. "If one of you is ill, he should send for the elders of the church and let them anoint him with oil in the name of the Lord and pray over him. The prayer of faith will save the sick man, and the Lord will raise him up again; and if he has committed any sins, he will be forgiven. So confess your sins to one another and pray for one another, and this will heal you." James 5:14-15 In my years as a pastor I welcomed the privilege of taking Holy Communion to the sick. I believed that I was taking the very life of Christ to them.

There is renewed interest in anointing the sick with oil. We are becoming more informed about the significance of anointing in the scriptures. In the Old Testament the word, anoint, is used 30 times in the New Testament 5 times. Anointed appears 80 times in the Old Testament and in the New Testament 3 times. When David was anointed as king, the priest used oil. Oil was also used for the anointing of priests to their office. It is in the New Testament that oil is used as a ministry to the sick. "And they cast out many devils and anointed with oil many that were sick and healed them." Mark 6:13

There is no magic in the oil. It is the Lord who heals, and it is in His name that the oil is applied to the sick. As a chaplain, I have anointed persons who were unconscious or so seriously ill that they were unable to make a verbal response but did respond with gestures. When I anointed with oil and the patient was unable to respond, I would ask the family to respond on behalf of the patient.

Another important aspect of the anointing with oil is that of confession of sin. The confession of faults is very important to complete healing. One of the things that create illness is guilt, and I believe that there can never be complete healing if guilt weighs heavily upon the patient. It can be said that confession is good for the soul and also for the body and mind.

The patient has the choice between wisdom and despair when confronting his illness. Wild Bill, a prisoner in a German concentration camp, made the choice for wisdom. Most prisoners thought Wild Bill had recently arrived in the camp because he seemed to have endless energy. Others knew that he had lived for six interminable years on the prison's starvation disease and in the disease-ridden barracks. Before his imprisonment Wild Bill lived in Warsaw's Jewish ghetto with his wife, three sons, and two daughters. Bill witnessed the Nazis shoot every member of his family. He begged the soldiers to kill him too rather than exile him to a concentration camp. Because he knew six languages and they needed a camp interpreter, they did not kill him.

Wild Bill tells how his attitude changed: "I had to decide right then whether to let myself hate the soldiers who had done this. It was an easy decision. I was a lawyer and in my practice I had seen what hate could do to people's minds and bodies. Hate had just killed the six people who mattered most to me in the world. I decided that I would spend the rest of my life, whether it was a few days or many years, loving every person I came in contact with." He poured out his love in six languages for eighteen hours a day reconciling arguments among the different nationalities in the camp. He moved from despair to wisdom.

Erik Erikson suggests that despair ordinarily begins with contempt of individuals, then encompasses institutions and finally leads to contempt of oneself. On the other hand, tragedy can lead to wisdom when it leads someone like Wild Bill to reconstruct the meaning of his life. Thus he determined to love every person I come in contact with and to be a camp reconciler. To construct such meaning one has to acknowledge one's loss and to forgive others and then to accept the fact that one's life is one's own responsibility.

The following prayer was found at the Ravensbruck death camp where 92,000 children and women died. It was scrawled on wrapping paper near a dead child.

"Lord, remember not only the men and women of good will but also those of ill will. Do not only remember the suffering they had inflicted on us; remember the fruits we have brought, thanks to this suffering: our comradeship, our loyalty, our humility, the courage, the generosity, and the greatness of hearts which has grown out of all this, and when they come to judgment, let all the fruit we have borne be their forgiveness."

Healing is found in many people at the final stage of life which Erikson calls the age of wisdom. Erikson emphasizes that wisdom is more like gratitude rather despair in rejecting one's later years of diminishment. It is the acceptance of one's own and only life cycle and of the people who have become significant to it…free of the wish that they should have been different, and an acceptance of the fact that one's life is one's own responsibility. Wisdom is being able to look back on your life and find how you have grown through everything. It is eliminating the wish that things should have been different. We call it the peace of God which passes all understanding. Even at the early stages of one's life when you exercised great power as an executive, you later learn that power always wears out those who wear the power.

At the turn of the 20th century it was believed that medical science would solve all the problems of the human body. Illness would be abolished. We know today that new medical problems are coming with new challenges: AIDS and cancer. The medical approach has added twenty years to the average life span during the last century. In the last fifty years the medical view of sickness has been changing. With the advance of psychiatry and the increased importance of chronic illness, medicine is taking a new look at the factors that cause disease. More hospitals have added Spiritual Care Departments to provide spiritual care for patients and staff.

Hans Selye writes in his book, The Stresses Of Life, that adrenal exhaustion can be caused by emotional tension, such as frustration or suppressed rage. He details how these emotional states affect the body chemistry in a negative way. Love, hope, faith, laughter, confidence, and the will-to-live produce positive changes. A member of our cancer support group says that he tells jokes all the time to make others laugh as well as himself. He's sure that laughter helps him in his struggle with cancer. Johnny Carson was a member of my Midshipman's Class during World War II. Like I was, he was commissioned as a naval officer. He was funny then. Then when he became famous, he brought lots of laughter to millions of people which I'm sure helped many to cope with illness.

God works in mysterious ways to change our negative attitudes to positive ones. When I was in Hiroshima, two months after the atomic bomb was dropped, I was standing in the midst of total destruction. In the distance I saw some Japanese children walking over the rubble towards me. I wondered where they came from. They were about six years old. When they got to where I was, they said, "Chocoletto! Chocoletto!" They had learned somehow that American servicemen had Hershey chocolate bars. I had none, but a strange experience happened to me. From the depths of my being came words that I had learned in Sunday school: "Jesus loves all the children of the world." Immediately my negative attitude about our former enemies changed into a positive one: "These are God's children too."

One day I was called to the intensive care unit to give Last Rites to a Shoshone Native American woman. There were 12 relatives in the room. I introduced myself and then said that I was a minister to the Sioux Indians in North Dakota. I said that the name of the Sunday school teacher was Mrs. Helen Wise Spirit. They thought that was a beautiful name and the patient's sister said: "The Sioux are noted for the beautiful names they give to their children." My mentioning of my work with the Sioux created a positive attitude towards me. I was no longer a stranger.

At another time I was called for the same reason for a woman from the Philippines. I told them that I was in Manila on their first

Independent Day on July 4, 1946 after their country was liberated by American military forces. They all smiled and thanked me. They said none of them had been born then except one. At that time she was just one year old. Again the common history enabled us to relate to one another.

Dr. Ana Aslan, one of Romania's leading endocrinologists, believes there is a direct connection between a robust will to live and the chemical balances in the brain. She states that we ought not to underestimate the capacity of the human mind and body to regenerate even when the prospects seem most wretched. Our life force may be the least understood force in the world.

Concerning the existence of life, it is true, even if in different ways, that God's omnipotence, God's workings, are present in it. Even in the being of the atom we come upon the mystery of the divine presence and power. Hence, there is absolutely no existence without mystery; therefore behind the form of being even that of a simple atom of hydrogen or of an electron, there lies the whole mystery of the Divine Omnipotence. In the spiritual realm of life God is the one great restorer of life.

Suppose your doctor wrote out a prescription after your latest checkup which said: "Here's a medication I want you to take. It will greatly lessen your chances of contracting at least half a dozen diseases that you become increasingly vulnerable to after the age of thirty-five." Would you get the prescription filled and then take it? "Well, there are at least half a dozen diseases that can be fended off or avoided altogether with the help of an appropriate exercise program. There are no absolute guarantees just as there are none where medications are concerned. The overwhelmingly evidence suggests that you'd be well advised to follow the prescription.

Another part of my health acronym for becoming well again is attitude. An open attitude allows you to listen to your doctor's advice about new medications. You essentially become a student of your doctor who is willing to share with you the best of his experience and knowledge. As you know, attitude is extremely critical in any type of illness. Studies show that with a positive attitude you fare much better in recovering from any type of illness. The members of our cancer support group affirm how beneficial it was for them to keep a positive attitude throughout their treatment. One of the reasons they come back to the group is because they gained knowledge and encouragement from the other members.

In the Bible we read: "A merry heart makes good medicine but a broken spirit dries the bones." Proverbs 17:22 Sir Francis Bacon called attention to the physiological characteristics of mirth. I believe all of us enjoyed the antics of Victor Borge on the piano. He had his audience in stitches with his zany actions. You always felt better after watching him on TV. Four hundred years ago Robert Burton quoted authorities for his observation that "humor purges the blood, making the body young, lively and fit for any manner of employment." Burton said that mirth is the principal engine for battering the walls of melancholy. Thomas Hobbes, philosopher, described laughter as a "passion of sudden glory.

I found the following quotations from a book I bought in 1946 when I was a naval officer. I had a great desire to learn about life and what the great thinkers had to say about it. Little did I realize that I would be quoting from it 65 years later. Immanuel Kant, another great philosopher in his "Critique of Pure Reason," wrote that laughter produces a feeling of health that makes up the gratification felt by us so that we reach the body through the soul and use the soul as the physician to the body. Sir William Osler, one of the greatest physicians ever known, wrote that laughter is the "music of the soul." The positive emotion of laughter has great power to heal the body in conjunction with a good sense of humor.

Allen Klein in his book, The Healing Power Of Humor, writes about the physiological effects of laughter. He quotes from the French philosopher, Voltaire, "The art of medicine consists of amusing the patient while nature cures the disease." The Greeks included a visit to the "home of the comedians" as part of their healing process, and the American Ojibwa Indian tribe had clown doctors perform antics to cure the sick. Dr. James Walsh, author of Laughter and Health, wrote that there seems no doubt that hearty laughter stimulates practically all the large organs.

Norman Cousins made the joyous discovery that ten minutes of belly-laughter had an anesthetic effect and would give him at least two hours of pain-free sleep. The Christian faith offers a perspective on life that urges the person not to take life too seriously, because it will be over, and many of the things we worry about either never happen or are not all that important.

A very important part of my acronym is spirituality. Faith in God does make a difference in our life especially when we are sick. God inspires people to help other people who have also been hurt by life. By helping others they protect themselves from the danger of loneliness. God makes some people want to become doctors and nurses, to spend days and nights of self-sacrificing concern with an intensity for which no money can compensate in the effort to sustain life and alleviate pain. God moves people to want to be medical researchers, to focus their intelligence and energy on the causes and possible cures for some of life's tragedies.

Everything you are had its origin in your mother's womb. Your body and soul were fashioned together according to the foreknowledge and wisdom of God. He knitted us in our mother's womb as it is recorded in the Bible. You were mostly blessed when you were a baby in the sacrament of Baptism.

Conclusion

We are called by God to care for the sick as well as to care for our own body as the temple of God. We are called by God to pray for the sick and to visit them so that they may become well again. The Apostle John wrote: "Beloved, I pray that all may go well with you and that you may be in health. I know it is well with your soul." 3 John 1:2 The Anglican Church as early as 130 adopted a report on healing: "Within the church...systems of healing based on the redemptive work of our Lord...all spring from a belief in the fundamental principle that the power to exercise spiritual healing is taught by Christ to be the natural heritage of Christian people who are living in fellowship with God and is part of the ministry of Christ through His Body the Church."[22] The resolution called for "a fuller understanding of the intimate connection between moral and spiritual disorders and mental and physical ills. It stresses ministry to the whole person. The bishops announced publicly that the anointing and the laying on of hands can have a direct effect on the body.

There is an old Arabian proverb which says: "He who has health has hope, and he who has hope has everything." Ralph Waldo Emerson wrote: "The first wealth is health."

The starting point is to become aware of the manner in which beliefs affect outcomes in many areas of one's personality and behavior. To listen carefully and attentively to the voices of suffering is the demanding challenge of the church. We can't remove the suffering, but we can help them find its deeper meaning for their lives.

---

22 A footnote to The Ministry of Healing Report-Resolution 163 of the Lamberth Conference-1930

Dr. Carl Jung told one of his patients: "You are suffering from a loss of faith in God and in a future life." The patient responded: "But, Dr. Jung, do you believe these doctrines are true?" Dr. Jung: "That is no business of mine. I am a doctor. I can only tell you that if you recover your faith, you will get well. If you don't, you won't." Recovery from a serious illness or accident provides an incentive to make a new beginning. Surviving a heart attack often results in a profound gratitude to the medical team and to God. The opportunity to begin anew is open to each one of us. God does allow U turns in our life! Let's make that turn to health now! God bless you and keep you well.

www.ingramcontent.com/pod-product-compliance
Lightning Source LLC
Chambersburg PA
CBHW070552290526
45790CB00002B/656